I0621230

Healthcare

Quality
for the Rest of Us

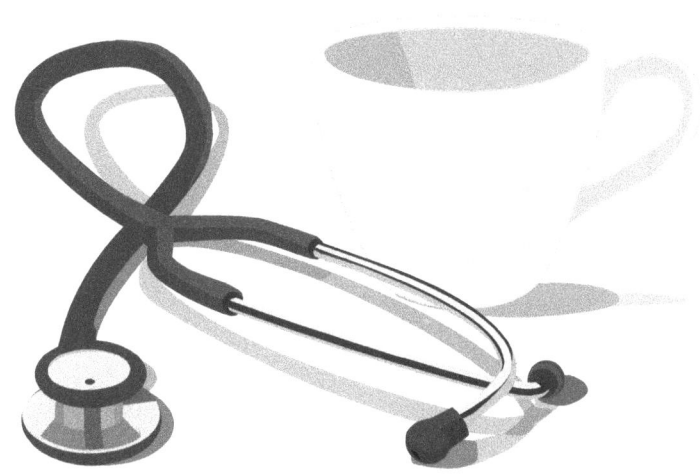

A Friendly Guide to Healthcare Quality Management

Gayle Porter RN CPHQ

ISBN: 978-1-957907-08-6 (Paperback)
ISBN: 978-1-957907-09-3 (Ebook)

Library of Congress Control Number: 2023944171

Any references to historical events, real people, or real places have been altered and fictionalized to protect the identities of those involved.

Book design by Stephen Porter.

E-book published by Porter Creative at Smashwords.

Porter Creative

3647 Oviedo

Brownsville TX 78520

www.portercreatives.com

Dedication

To the healthcare professionals who see potential in every roadblock, and the patients who remind us why such improvements matter.

Acknowledgements

This book would not exist without the knowledge and dedication of my husband, Stephen Porter. You have my immense gratitude for your editing, beautiful design, formatting, guidance, patience and encouragement. Thank you for taking the time to help me translate the field of healthcare quality, and for your love and friendship as we worked together.

Thanks to the community and subscribers at the PorterQI website and the Quality for the Rest of Us podcast for your support from the earliest beginning.

I would like to thank Betsy Serrao for introducing me to this professional field and mentoring me. I have met many professionals who did not have a Betsy in their lives to show them the ropes, and I am forever grateful for the time, wisdom, and patience that you invested in me. You helped me understand so much more than job skills or professional trends; you helped me understand people and coached me to strengthen the moral compass that guides my work.

Thank you to Mary Randall for being an incredible leader and source of wisdom in quality improvement and abstraction. Your calm and caring leadership was an inspiring example, and you offered fresh challenges with optimism and creativity. I am grateful for your influence on my life.

Thank you to Pete Aguirre for showing me how important it is to listen to patients and colleagues for solutions, and for demonstrating how significant those simple innovations could be for real people. Special thanks to Sonia Ortiz-Leon for introducing me to patient safety and for listening to my crazy ideas while we shared an office, and to Honeylane DeSosa for showing me the amazing world of infection prevention.

Thanks to my friend and colleague, Anne Dempsey, who encouraged me to write because she believes in the message of healthcare quality with such inspiring passion. Thank you for dedicating so much of your life to mentoring others, and for showing me what empathy beyond-the-bedside looks like in real life.

Thank you, Jennifer Sipert, for being a role model for servant-leadership in healthcare quality, and for reminding me how amazing it is to see positive transformation in healthcare.

I'm also grateful to the National Association for Healthcare Quality (NAHQ) for developing education and standards that would build structure and professionalism into my career.

Warm thanks to my family for believing in this project. Special thanks to my children, Nathaniel and Elizabeth, for cheering me on and reminding me why this all matters.

I could not begin to name all of the leaders, friends and colleagues who have taught and encouraged me in this profession, but I am grateful to know you and to share this purpose of improving healthcare for our beloved patients and communities together.

Thank you to my readers, who gave me a reason to write. To every professional who is still figuring out how to improve healthcare, your zeal for better outcomes not only affects the numbers on data sheets, but it improves the real lives of patients in their moments of vulnerability. Thank you for being compassionate and curious, and for joining me in this amazing profession to improve healthcare for real people.

From Gayle Porter

The host of the podcast Quality for the Rest of Us

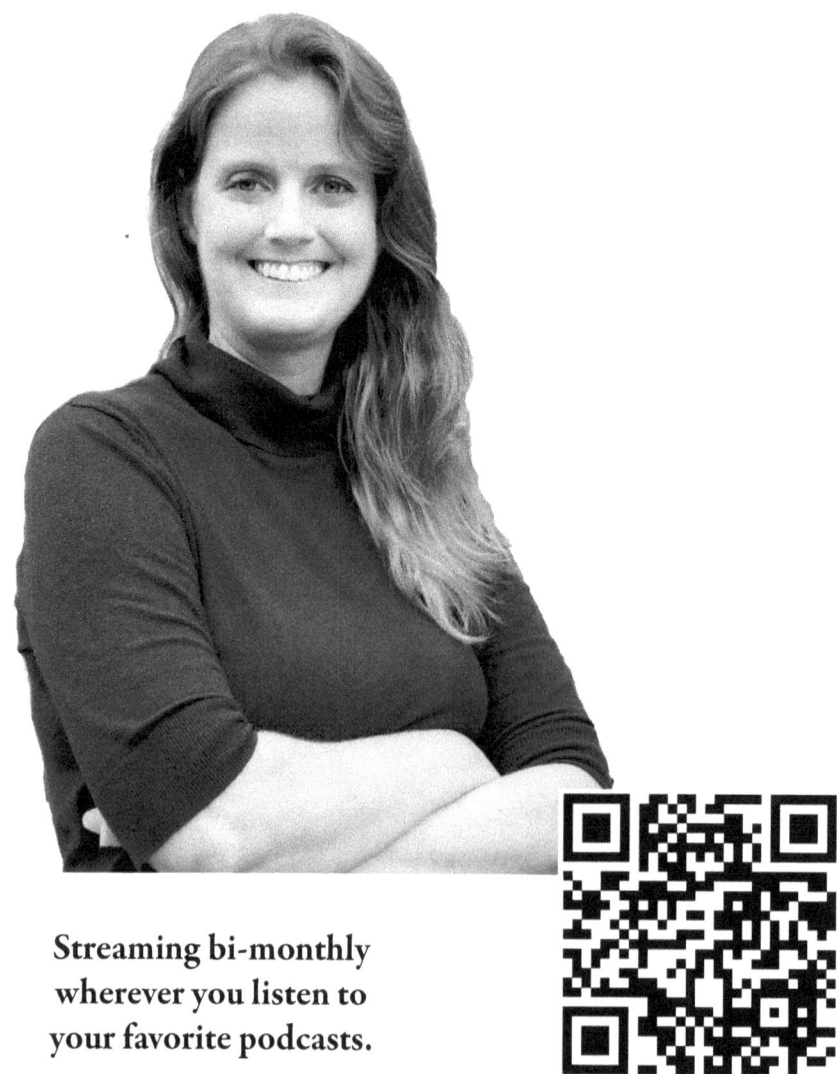

Streaming bi-monthly
wherever you listen to
your favorite podcasts.

Table of Contents

Introduction

When I interviewed for a job as a quality analyst years ago, I was not entirely sure what the job entailed—I just knew that I needed to make a change and that I liked studying and solving mysteries. As a child, I walked around with a pencil behind my ear and a notepad in my hands looking for something "mysterious" and pretending to be a very serious detective. As a nurse, I loved investigating a patient's condition: from tracing "clues" in their history, to recording "evidence" from labs and vital signs, to the final step of reporting my findings in a CSI-style summary for the rounding physician.

But I was not entirely sure being behind a desk in the Quality Department was going to fit my detective paradigm, and stepping into the job did not alleviate that anxiety. On my first day of work in the Quality Department, my new boss showed me a tracker that listed patient charts pending "abstraction," and I understood that I needed to fill out electronic forms about their care to keep up with that tracker. I was informed that if my boss saw the color red in that list, I would be in trouble for not keeping up, but I had no clue where the information went or what it was for—and that pretty much summarizes the expectations I had for my job as a Quality Improvement (QI) professional when I first started. My first QI mystery to solve was just to answer the question "why?" Why did healthcare quality exist at all?

After I answered that question, I fell in love with my job. I have worked with more than one hundred hospitals to improve their patient care through quality projects, and I frequently receive questions from nurses and other healthcare professionals asking about the work we do in quality, wondering where they can make a difference to improve patient care. If you are like me and enjoy looking for ways to improve processes, get a thrill from the detective work of digging through patients' charts, or get excited about studying new things with a variety of other departments, then QI is a place that can really light-up your skills and interests. If you are in a QI role currently but want to increase your confidence, or simply wish to learn some innovative ways to apply QI tools at your hospital, I want to warmly welcome you to the practical ideas in this book.

About This Book

This book is a conversation where I can share my experiences, mistakes, and discoveries, and identify key resources for success in QI. Through this book I hope to answer questions like:

- How did QI become a part of healthcare?
- What types of data are commonly used by QI professionals?
- How does the Nursing Process apply to QI?
- What are useful tools out of the many resources available?
- What are some helpful organizations that provide research and policies?
- How to make sense of the abstraction of data?
- What are the key organizations for reporting data?
- What is the process of submitting CDAC audits to CMS for validation?
- Who are some of the collaborative partners in QI and how are the Clinical Documentation Improvement (CDI) team, Informatics, and Coding teams involved?
- What is the role of the Healthcare QI Professional as it continues to evolve and standardize?

Throughout the book, I have included helpful **Tech Tips** with details about using technology in QI, as well as **Resource Lists** with the

locations of helpful organizations and resources. The
Featured Tool boxes include suggestions based on my experience trying
to solve healthcare mysteries in data and documentation. And the
Example Problem boxes will present some case studies to show Quality
Improvement in action.

I have written this book for those without clinical experience,
individuals who are just starting in a new position in quality, and experienced quality professionals who wish to enhance their QI skills: all with
the goal of improving patient care because whether you are clinical or
not, every facet of healthcare is ultimately geared toward the lives of our
patients.

Disclaimers

To protect privacy and maintain compliance with the Healthcare Insurance Portability and Accountability Act (HIPAA), all examples were
taken from de-identified locations and projects or were invented by the
author to reflect real-life experiences.

This book does not serve as a final authority on the topic but
provides information on some of the resources that were useful in my
professional experiences. Information provided is current as of publication, but this field is quickly evolving: Websites, measures, and best
practices may change. Please visit *https://porterqi.com* for up-to-date
information on this text, and refer to primary sources for legal and
regulatory updates.

Chapter 1
What is Healthcare Quality Improvement?

What is the purpose of Healthcare Quality Improvement (QI) exactly? And what does it mean to have quality "for the rest of us"? I will first define and explore these terms and provide a brief history of the field because it helps to have some context for the topics discussed later in the book. I will also share how to learn more about the Certified Professional in Healthcare Quality (CPHQ) certification and describe Patient Safety as a separate and growing field. Like many fields, QI has a lot of technical language and complicated acronyms—but the concepts are simple. That simplicity is what I focus on in this text because QI does not need to be complicated and unapproachable. It is meant to foster better communication and improve patient care across the greater healthcare team. Success is measured by actual, tangible improvement in care, not by a flashy vocabulary.

What Is The Purpose?

At the most basic level, Healthcare QI uses evidence to improve patient care. The evidence is primarily taken from medical record, and the improvement of care happens at all levels from direct patient care to the executive board. At every one of these levels, there is a lot of change and risk in healthcare, and for many facilities one of the first goals is to be resilient, adjusting to change without diminishing patient care. Effective QI can help mitigate some of the risk involved in healthcare, both for the patients and all levels of staff. So how does QI affect patient care in practical terms?

To answer that question, we need to take a look at what patient care is supposed to look like, what it actually looks like, and why there is a gap between the two.

The Ideal Patient Experience

My first clinical experience was at a prestigious teaching hospital, where patient care was constantly adjusted based on the best practices informed by the most up-to-date research. Nursing staff coordinated treatment with a team of skilled specialists in nutrition, therapy, and other departments. Physicians collaborated with nursing staff, and the clinical team carefully scheduled time to educate, treat, and discuss care with the patient. The patient was the most important person, and we had to respect the patient's schedule to avoid delays in treatment. The hospital attracted the best healthcare professionals at every level. The patients I met said their care was personal, purposeful, and efficient, and I was impressed and humbled with the care I witnessed.

One day during my clinical experience, my nursing instructor abruptly stopped us in the hallway and introduced us to an environmental services (EVS) employee cleaning a patient's room. Her name was Lydia. My professor said, "this is the most important member of the hospital care team." My professor eyed each of us warily before she continued: "Without Lydia, the next patient would be fighting resistant infections rather than getting better and going home. Lydia is highly trained to clean effectively and sanitize the room and equipment. The cleaning sprays must be timed for maximum germ control, and the delicate screens on the machines can break down if the wrong cleaners are used. Make sure you respect her work and say thank you to the environmental services team—because your job would be useless without them." Then she turned on her heel and marched down the hallway as we all said "thank you" to Lydia and trailed after our instructor sheepishly.

The Reality

Fast forward a couple of years and I found myself trying to join the workforce after a recession. Everyone in my nursing class had difficulty finding work without prior experience. We all lost our internships. Hospitals were struggling, and many of them experienced budget cuts. When I found work, it was at a community hospital in one of the most impoverished counties in the nation. My preceptor described long-lasting problems, and budget constraints resulted in delays to replace broken equipment. I also discovered that each monthly staff meeting included announcements that nursing staff would be picking up a new duty previously managed by a supporting department: The environmental services department could no longer remove linens at discharge. Nursing would make the bed for new admissions and take over sanitizing equipment and removing garbage.

I remembered Lydia. These tasks required training and consistency, but the nurses were unaccustomed to monitoring the kill-time of cleaning sprays or determining which sanitizer was less likely to melt the IV pump's screen. We were also dealing with an electronic record that demanded instant gratification akin to a timed video game—and if we did not keep up with it, harm could come to our patients, whom we had not seen for most of the shift due to the burgeoning demands of documentation and extra tasks. As I listened to my patients, they described care that was impersonal, stating that they believed their own nurse could not remember their names. Little by little, infections and pressure ulcers began to increase, and we began to rush the environmental services team to clean faster and faster to accommodate our admissions and transfers.

At first, I was disappointed with some of the reactive responses to adverse events: Nurses on my team were sometimes counseled or written up for being the "origin" of hospital-acquired incidents, even though the changes to our role and cleaning process may have directly related to the uptick in infections and pressure ulcers. There had to be a better solution, but the boardroom and the bedside did not seem to understand each other.

Our hospital was not alone in this struggle to prevent harm and provide safe and effective care. The Institute of Medicine (IOM) issued a national agenda for reducing medical errors, which were reported to be the third leading cause of death in the nation by 2019.[1] This news came with corresponding changes to an increasingly technical, yet unsupported, nursing workforce.[2] The pandemic of 2020-2022 only deepened the problems as nearly 6% of baby-boomers retired from the workforce permanently, meaning most of the older, most experienced healthcare workers left, never to return. Hospitals faced massive staffing shortages, and burnout rates soared. My personal experience showed that when nurses complained about their role or workload, those complaints often started fruitless arguments, or worse, an extra audit was introduced to investigate the complaint. More paperwork. When did we have time for an audit when we were already drowning?

What on earth happened? Was the quality of care I witnessed in nursing school just a utopia, or was it possible to have "quality for the rest of us?"

Using Quality to Bridge the Gap

This type of situation is what prompted me, along with many professionals, to look for better ways to communicate about the issues that are sometimes quite clear at the bedside but seem to be invisible in the boardroom. While staff complaints did not elicit change, a detailed spreadsheet could show relationships about the best use of our resources. I guess that was when it first started to click: When I could measure a problem and show a solution that could cut costs, decrease harm, or reduce waste, I could see real change occur at the bedside—

1   Kohn, L.T.; Corrigan, J.M.; Donaldson, M.S. (Eds.) (2000). *To Err is Human: Building a Safer Health System*. National Academies Press.

2   Anderson, J.G.; Abrahamson, K. (2017). Your Health Care May Kill You: Medical Errors. *Stud Health Technol Inform* 234, 13-17.

patients could get better. I just needed to use the data to communicate what our patients needed.

Using data to improve care is the purpose of Healthcare QI. It is always about the patient, and QI continuously evolves because the needs of patients change. So we trained on sanitation and updated the par-stock allocation of cleaning supplies to make them readily available. We also reduced the detail and frequency of required assessments to cut down on the digital burden of documentation for nursing, which allowed more time to sanitize properly. None of us wanted to be scrubbing down IV pumps, but at least we could do it well, and it reduced the number of infections for our patients—that part always felt good. It became a task that we could take pride in, rather than an unsupported, "extra" burden. We were flexible, and we learned from it.

While QI projects are based on patient needs and can be highly individualized, there are still some consistent methods and workflows to help us study problems. This workflow begins with data analysis to identify problems, and then we carefully design projects and measure change using quality tools. In addition, QI professionals may conduct research, provide education, discuss outcomes with medical committees and executive boards, and report findings to regulatory organizations who share it with the public. The public reporting of data and its effect on financial reimbursement can be stressful, but it also increases executive support for QI projects. The QI professional can use data to show how patient care is more important to a healthcare organization's bottom line than any other metric.

Looking back, some of the greatest assets at the teaching hospital were that their executive team created a culture that put the patient first. They understood that the business of healthcare is more than a business that deals in health. It is a business that is designed to care, and caring leads to better health — which includes not just the patient, but valuing each member of the healthcare team. I will never forget that Lydia from environmental services possessed unique qualifications that are invaluable to the patient. She cared for the patient as much the highest-rated physician, and because of her care, the hospital had fewer hospital-acquired infections, which helped their bottom-line. This type of culture is literally priceless, and yet its return on investment leads to significant financial rewards.

Caring for others doesn't require a massive budget. The size of a hospital does not decide the quality of care, but the people and processes have a tremendous effect. And when I thought about it, I realized that that research hospital had to pin down the best solutions to the same problems everyone else had, and they had developed their culture of caring from evidenced-based studies – but our community hospital could reap the benefit of all their research if we could just translate those solutions into bite-sized ones that met local needs, and the answers for how that translation could happen was somewhere in the patient data. The purpose of QI is always to take this all-encompassing data, analyze it, and present evidence-based, culture-improving solutions for the best possible healthcare individual patients can receive in whatever medical situation they are facing.

This book shares a lot of evidence-based practices, but the real-life examples focus on practical solutions that can make a big difference at any hospital, regardless of the number of beds or size of the Quality Department. To provide first-rate patient care at every hospital, regardless of the budget, is to provide "quality for the rest of us." To value every member of the team, regardless of the prestige of their title, is to provide "quality for the rest of us." And training each new quality professional to communicate with data, bridging the gap between the boardroom and the bedside? That is "quality for the rest of us."

So where did QI get its start, and how do we know its principles will lead to the outcomes we're looking for? The history of QI was birthed out of tough decisions and significant changes to society, including wars, technical revolutions, and even pandemics. And what better metaphors could be used to describe today's healthcare system? Surely, if we can learn how quality was maintained in the very worst of times, it can help us provide better care in the present. If we're talking about the nuts and bolts of this industry, it literally came about from the nuts and bolts of manufacturing. Some of the first examples of QI practices that we'll look at come from Japanese manufacturing companies and the oil industry.

A Brief History

I inherited a large cedar chest from my grandmother that once served as her "hope chest" but later served as a memory-keeper for anything my grandma thought would be nice to remember. It is stuffed with letters and pictures, keepsakes, and some of the documents are in foreign languages. There are old yearbooks from my grandparent's high school, signed with quotes and paragraphs challenging them to be of good character as they graduate. I have barely scratched the surface of exploring this treasure trove of family history, but whenever I have the chance to put on my detective hat and look through these memories, I see so many connections between the choices my grandparents made in high school and the way our family is today; looking at our family history shows me what it means to be a part of my family.

In my new QI job, I found myself asking: What does it mean to be a part of the QI "family"? There were so many differences from bedside care, yet it was so methodical. So I am going to dust off a fascinating section of history to show how a QI professional thinks about problems and share how this role was created in the first place — kind of like dusting off a high school yearbook from my grandparent's generation. Who had the idea of measuring stuff, writing quality standards, and developing these methods? While I wish I could give a thorough family history of the field, this historical summary will be quite brief, highlighting only the methods that are most critical to understanding the role today.

Manufacturing

There was a sudden change during the Industrial Revolution from buying products from a local craftsman to large-scale mass production in factories. The development of factories dramatically increased the speed and efficiency of production, while decreasing the cost and time spent creating products, but mass production had also caused problems with product quality that could affect the product's reputation negatively. There was a new need to ensure that purchased factory goods were safe, reliable, and of good quality.[3] For example, John D. Rockefeller developed the Standard Oil company in the 1870s, which originally advertised "standardized" kerosene that was reliable and would not set fire to homes; unstable kerosene could explode and had caused entire homes to be lost.[4] Rockefeller's assurance of having a standardized product led to his eventual monopolization of kerosene production, then oil processing, and finally gasoline production. This type of standardization was a fairly new idea in the business world at that time, but it became clear very quickly that customers wanted it.

There was also a massive shift caused by the World Wars with troops returning home, women entering and leaving factory jobs, and economies rebuilding around the world. Amidst these turbulent changes, there was an opportunity to review safety and make changes to manufacturing, since so many other changes needed to occur anyway. By 1947, The International Organization for Standardization (ISO) was established as a non-governmental organization in Geneva, Switzerland to promote the development of standards in production. Today, ISO certification can be obtained by organizations in a variety of fields, from automotive manufacturing to healthcare.

The practical aspects of QI accelerated with post-World War II factories in Japan, where the economy was in shambles after their defeat by the Allied nations, and the need to rebuild almost from scratch made it possible to invent a new, better process in manufacturing. A key name to remember from this era is Dr. William Edwards Deming, who was an engineer and statistician (among other things). While working

---

3   American Society for Quality (2022). Quality Resources. Retrieved on Jan. 27, 2022, from https://asq.org/quality-resources/standards-101#iso.

4   Reams, P.; Magan, R. (Directors) (2012). *The Men Who Built America* [Film]. The History Channel.

for the U.S. Census Bureau during Japan's Restoration, he presented a seminar on statistical process control in Japan and developed a collaboration with the Union of Japanese Scientists and Engineers. His ideas for applying statistics to analyze and improve factory production led to an invitation for him to travel to Japan in the 1950s to work with business leaders on improving the quality of their post-war manufacturing process.[5] He believed that reliable outcomes could be achieved by minimizing variation — by studying the errors and mistakes that varied from the norm, they could find ways to reduce the number of errors and "standardize" the outcome: a perfect final product. Deming's quality principles were applied to many fields, and over the course of his career he developed methods of continuous improvement, efficiency, and quality control. His ideas were quite successful and helped post-war Japan's economy to recover and prosper. By the 1980s, Japan entered a season of global manufacturing dominance by reducing mistakes and product defects (variation), while increasing efficiency and resilience.[6] Deming's principles of QI are also called the "Toyota Way" after the Japanese auto manufacturer that made them famous.

Applications in Healthcare

While the success of Deming's ideas in Japan resulted in multiple derivatives of the Toyota Way, the original is most applicable to healthcare because of its emphasis on respect for people and their capabilities. The ability of individuals to take pride in their work and practice continuous improvement on an individual level is an inspiring method of management. Through these principles and success stories, Deming came to be considered the "father" of Healthcare QI, even though he worked with machine production rather than caring for the sick.

---

5   Tague, Nancy (2005). *The Quality Toolbox* (2nd edition). ASQ Quality Press.

6   *William Edwards Deming: The Father of Quality Management* (Jan. 27, 2022). Creative Safety Supply. Retrieved on April 5, 2022 from https://creativesafetysupply. com/articles/william-edwards-deming-the-father-of-quality-management/.

More recently (and similar to Deming's principles), Six Sigma has become an important name in healthcare quality with a set of principles devoted to reducing variation or flaws in a process. The Sigma score itself is a statistical measure of defect-free products in each batch. The Six Sigma folks use a process known as DMAIC: Define, Measure, Analyze, Improve, Control; this method defines the problem and has a period of data collection and study prior to introducing any changes. After changes are made, the next step is to control for variation and look for future opportunities for improvement. Six Sigma also empha-sizes having clear roles and titles for the members of the team and uses purposeful review to improve processes and reduce mistakes. I noticed that some QI professionals carry certifications like "Six Sigma Green Belt" or "Six Sigma Black Belt," for example, to indicate their training level and role in the Six Sigma method, and it is helpful to know what the title means. For example, a green belt might work in analysis and implementation and a black belt might work in project management and delegation.

Curiously, I found that these manufacturing-centered QI methods are quite similar to the Nursing Process, which is itself quite similar to the scientific method. This realization was a bit of a relief to me when I was new to the field. Throughout the history of nursing, there are plenty of stories of nurses cleaning up entire facilities, improving patient care, and reforming systems, and it makes sense. For example, Mary Breck-inridge identified a problem with reaching Appalachian patients. She determined that she could reach them on horseback, but once she saw patients and assessed the population's needs, she discovered she would need more staff as well. She came up with a new solution and set-up mountain clinics staffed by the Frontier Nursing Service — a workforce she established in 1925 to meet the healthcare needs of patients living in remote areas of Kentucky.[7] Nurses like Florence Nightingale,[8] Dorothea Dix,[9] Alice Fisher,[10] and Clara Barton[11] have similar stories of reforming healthcare to improve patient care for a specific population using a method of assessment, problem identification, planning, treatment, and re-assessment.

When I trained in QI and learned the various methods of problem identification and data analysis, I kept exclaiming, "Oh, so it's just like the Nursing Process?" Investing time to learn the acronyms of different QI methods made me sound more professional, but I found that just a basic knowledge of the Nursing Process provided the framework of how to prepare QI projects and improve quality for patients. Chapter 3: Project Management covers using the Nursing Process as a guide to QI project management with real-life examples and projects to illustrate the steps. Even without a nursing background, a high school knowledge of the scientific method (ask a question, study a change, measure what happened) is enough to understand the concepts.

The practice of continuous improvement is somewhat native to nurses, though, because of the nursing care plan: Each nursing diagnosis in the care plan requires constant reassessment, and wherever a deficit is found, an intervention is required. If my patient is at-risk for skin break-

7   Wells, Rosemary (2002). *Mary on Horseback: Three mountain stories.* Puffin.

8   The History Channel (2022). "Women's History: Florence Nightingale." A&E Television Networks. Retrieved Aug. 30, 2022, from https://www.history.com/topics/womens-history/florence-nightingale-1.

9   Norwood, A.R. (2017). "Dorothea Dix." National Women's History Museum. Retrieved Aug. 30, 2022 from https://www.womenshistory.org/education-resources/biographies/dorothea-dix.

10   The American Nurses Association (n.d.). "The History of the American Nurses Association." About ANA. Retrieved Feb. 23, 2022, from https://www.nursingworld.org/ana/about-ana/history.

11   The American National Red Cross (2022). "Clara Barton: Visionary Leader and Founder of the American Red Cross." Our History. Retrieved Aug. 30, 2022, from https://www.redcross.org/about-us/who-we-are/history/clara-barton.html.

down and has nutritional deficits, a nutrition consult would be called and special skin ointments would be applied to protect the patient's skin from damage—but I would continue to measure the patient's caloric intake and skin condition as long as they are at risk: There is no point in patient care when I would say to my patient, "It doesn't look like you need anything." This is just another way of thinking about continuous improvement — the job is never finished, because even if nothing is immediately wrong, I would always be looking for areas of risk, trying to anticipate the next potential problem. And since healthcare does not "own" QI, I have found helpful resources in other fields including business, marketing, and computer science because they are all using the same QI principles.

As previously mentioned, this is a short history of highlights, but there are many opportunities for further study. To learn more about the history of QI as a field, or for a detailed guide to analytical quality tools, I highly recommend *The Quality Toolbox* by Nancy R. Tague.[12] I was on a tight budget when I first started in my QI position, and additional funding to pursue training was not available, but Tague's book was one of the most cost-effective sources I have found for becoming a fluent QI professional. One feature in her book is that it showed how to apply tools for certain types of problems and how to display the data in a way that helps others see the problem. If I had a process problem, for example, there were certain tools that were effective to find process problems and communicate them to others. I heard about *The Quality Toolbox* from a recommended reading list while studying for the Certified Professional in Healthcare Quality (CPHQ) exam, and it was pretty life-changing to be able to communicate what I could see at the bedside in a way that made sense to the business leaders at the hospital. There are other comprehensive sources available through some of the healthcare quality organizations mentioned in "Chapter 4: Simple Tools," but if I had to choose a favorite, *The Quality Toolbox* would take first place.

---

12   Tague, Nancy (2005). *The Quality Toolbox* (2nd edition). ASQ Quality Press.

CPHQ Certification

The CPHQ certification mentioned above can currently be achieved without prior experience and without a nursing license. The exam preparation covers very practical topics for anyone working in Healthcare QI and was immensely helpful in my practical work. I was inspired by the reading while I studied for the exam and used many of the tools and materials in my job. I highly recommend the whole experience of studying for the CPHQ exam and maintaining current knowledge of the field with the National Association for Healthcare Quality (NAHQ), who offers the certification. To learn more about the CPHQ Exam, visit the NAHQ's website: *https://nahq.org/certification/certified-professional-healthcare-quality/*.

Patient Safety: Similar but Different

The CPHQ exam currently includes a Patient Safety component, but there are also separate certifications offered exclusively in Patient Safety. For example, the Institute for Healthcare Improvement (IHI) offers a Certified Professional in Patient Safety (CPPS) certification.[13] Patient Safety focuses on preventing patient harm and may be part of a separate department in a hospital, or it could be a combined role with a QI position.

In my first QI position, I shared an office with the Patient Safety Coordinator, so it was literally impossible to avoid learning about the process and tools of Patient Safety. I attended all the webinars, volunteered to teach topics like Alarm Fatigue at the nursing skills fair, and served on the adverse events committee. I complained bitterly when I had to listen to webinars about grandmothers getting the wrong joint operation while the Patient Safety Coordinator listened to national

---

13   The Institute for Healthcare Improvement (April 14, 2022). "CPPS: Certified Professional in Patient Safety." Education. Retrieved Oct. 10, 2022, from http://www.ihi.og/education/cpps-certified-professional-in-patient-safety/pages/default.aspx.

updates by The Joint Commission (TJC) — but I am grateful for the experience today, and it definitely helped to see the Patient Safety methods in my CPHQ study guide put into practice.

The Patient Safety professional pays special attention to reviewing "near misses," or times when harm almost occurred, and they manage the Root Cause Analysis (RCA) and mandatory reporting if harm occurs. Every patient fall is reported to the Patient Safety professional, and they are tasked with creating an "environment of patient safety" within the facility, where everyone is willing to talk about how to keep patients safe and discuss problems that could cause harm. Safety guidelines may come from a variety of sources based on research findings, but the key player in leading Patient Safety is The Joint Commission (TJC), which sets reporting standards and establishes quality measures to prevent patient harm, like the National Patient Safety Goals. The Patient Safety professional takes these measures and is tasked with educating staff and reviewing the medical record for the Risk Manager in legal reviews. They work up cases for hospital-acquired injuries, if they occur, and often work closely with Infection Prevention to review potential hospital-acquired infections. The Patient Safety role carries a heavy load during surveys for hospital accreditation as they report on policies, procedures, and staff education focused on preventing patient harm. It is a broad field and studying for the CPHQ exam was a good way to start learning the methods and tools used in Patient Safety projects.

Many QI professionals will find themselves helping other departments, and it is a good opportunity to learn. For example, I learned about Infection Prevention while sorting reports in the computer for our busy Infection Prevention specialist, but when she asked me to help on her infection committee and demonstrated the use of a Failure Modes and Effects Analysis (FMEA) QI tool, I was able to see how a tool from my specialty could be applied in a live project. Needless to say, opportunities to cross-over and help colleagues can be valuable for QI professional development.

The next chapter focuses on the practical application of the history and theories we have discussed so far. Now that we know that one of the key founders of Healthcare QI was a statistician, it is time to look at data — because QI is not theoretical, it is inherently practical and should be based on data.

We will talk about why data matters, different types of data, how to pull data from the medical record and other sources, ways of organizing it, and how to use it to find and track problems.

Chapter 2
Data Analysis

As a nurse, I have a love-hate relationship with data. Sometimes, data can be the silver bullet that reveals the source of a complex problem, and other times, it seems to dehumanize patient care to the point that we no longer "see" our patients—just zeroes and ones in the matrix of the Electronic Medical Record (EMR). But without the data, we risk missing out on issues that affect our real patients. There are giant servers all over the nation holding multiple terabytes of patient data, and within these storage banks lie clues that could pull back the curtain on problems for individual patients, facilities, and entire populations. But interacting with this data introduces our personal bias and human fallibility. If it were so easy to mold the data into perfect solutions, we would have done it already. So, how do we interact with data without either neglecting the human side or skewing the numbers with our personal perspectives?

But data does not have to be so scary. There are parallels between data analytics and nursing, and a combination of nursing and data analysis can be especially beneficial to patient care. For example, let's take an aspect of nursing that we're all familiar with: taking vital signs. When I measure vital signs (temperature, pulse, respirations, blood pressure, pain score) and enter these numerical values into a chart, it is a type of hard data displayed on a flowsheet. These numbers are used to represent the health or dysfunction of multiple organs, which the human body depends on for survival. But how do we know what those numbers mean? The benchmark of what is normal for vital signs is based on previous knowledge and research of what is healthy (the normal limits), and without previous research we would not know if our patients had "good" or "bad" numbers.

Dysfunction in one organ affects the whole body and can make a patient "feel" ill. How the patient feels is often represented by a subjective component in the vitals (pain) with tailored parameters and a description of what is an acceptable level of pain. Since most patients come to the hospital with a complaint of pain, and not that their heart rate is too fast, we know that this subjective data can reveal a lot of important information about a problem. The human body has a massive amount of complex data, and vital signs are critical starting points in narrowing down the issues that might be affecting patient health; abnormalities in vital signs offer key clues into a patient's overall condition and risk.

Likewise, the health of a healthcare facility providing patient care is a complex system, and dysfunction in one element affects the whole system. Often, that dysfunction is expressed in subjective complaints from patients, staff, and other stakeholders. While the complaints can seem unrelated to patient care (like budgetary issues or staff burnout), the business of a healthcare facility is patient care, and if the business is experiencing pain, it is a good idea to start with what keeps the business alive and check the healthcare quality vital signs. The vital signs for healthcare quality include: 1) existing research, 2) raw facility data, and 3) patient tracers or case studies. (*see Table 2.1*)

Any abnormalities, such as research findings that are contrary to expectations or current practice (outside normal limits), like a batch of patients who experienced delays on the surgical ward, offer critical clues to the state of healthcare quality at a facility. These three sources of data serve as the Quality Improvement (QI) vital signs, so to speak, because they provide specific answers to clinical quality problems.

TABLE 2.1 FEATURED TOOL: QUALITY VITALS	
QUALITY DATA	**NURSING DATA**
Existing Research	Normal limits for temperature, pulse, respirations, and blood pressure
Raw Data	Recorded levels of patient's temperature, pulse, respirations, and blood pressure
Patient Tracers / Case Studies	Pain assessment

As an example, when a code sepsis protocol was initiated to help my facility meet the CMS Severe Sepsis and Septic Shock core measure,[1] we found that the obstetrics wing of the hospital was calling about three sepsis alerts per week. This result was much higher than we expected, and I was asked to investigate. We thought it might be human error because the nurses in obstetrics work with "otherwise healthy" patients, and they perhaps misunderstood the infection screening—or maybe the normal signs of labor skewed the sepsis assessment? The existing research did not mention obstetrics as a high-risk population, and our coding data only showed about one patient discharge with severe sepsis in the last 90 days from the obstetrics ward. In fact, globally most sepsis patients were supposed to be found in the Emergency Room or the Intensive Care Unit based on the coding data.

However, when we went to the bedside it became apparent that these patients were really sick, teetering on the edge of septic shock.

---

1   The Centers for Medicare and Medicaid Services (2022). "IQR Measures: Severe Sepsis and Septic Shock Management Bundle." QualiltyNet. Retrieved March 10, 2022, from https://qualitynet.cms.gov/inpatient/iqr/measures.

But if they were truly sick, how did we miss it? Was this a new thing, or had we missed it all along? The new sepsis alerts prompted us to look at each patient as a case study and conduct patient tracers. None of them came through the ED or transferred to the ICU and most patients were managed over the phone and coded with a mild infection rather than sepsis due to their rapid recovery—by the time the physician came on-site to see them, they looked much better after treatment. Our review showed that the obstetric sepsis alerts were accurate, even though the existing literature did not discuss it.

So how did we miss it then?

We examined community health demographics and found that sepsis incidence was higher in our predominantly Hispanic community overall, and more recent studies have reported a higher incidence of maternal complications among Hispanic women – particularly if they were diabetic. But without existing data, we had no idea it was an issue.[2]

Once the obstetric sepsis trend was confirmed in our maternal population, we found that coding of severe sepsis was limited because the local infection was often documented at discharge rather than severe sepsis. We believed the number of incidents went unnoticed because the obstetric unit did not generally call an alert for their maternal patients and they typically recovered quickly without a transfer to the ICU.

Smart Catch!

As a result, the quality department delivered a "smart catch award" to the obstetric nurses whose timely assessment and delivery of sepsis interventions saved the lives of our obstetric patients. As they received their rewards, the nurses reported how these patients had screened positive for sepsis, and they started a fluid bolus right away. Then, as the

---

2   Leonard, S.A.; Main, E.K.; Scott, K.A.; Profit, J.; Carmichael, S.L. (2019). Racial and ethnic disparities in severe maternal morbidity prevalence and trends. *Ann Epidemiol*(33): 30-36. Retrieved March 10, 2022, from https://pubmed.ncbi.nlm.nih.gov/30928320/.

fluid was going into the patient, their blood pressure started to drop. The sepsis screening had worked, and the treatment was just in time to preserve their vital organs. Our facility started a collaboration with the obstetric physician committee to improve sepsis prevention at the clinic level as well as in the hospital, and community education programs were initiated to teach women about preventing infection during pregnancy. A new perinatal resuscitation training program was introduced for critical care nurses, and maternal sepsis became a population-based benchmark for the sepsis program. Once the problem was identified and coding of sepsis severity became more accurate, the national centers for research had a spike in maternal sepsis codes to examine and new national quality measures were created to address healthcare disparities and maternal complications, including a unique CMS maternal sepsis screening to provide better guidance on interpreting signs and symptoms of sepsis under the condition of labor.[3]

There is just one thing: Without reviewing all three data sources, including the existing research presented by CMS, raw data on sepsis alerts, and case studies on obstetric sepsis alerts, these patients could have remained hidden. We were ready to re-educate and write-up nurses who were erroneously calling sepsis alerts rather than award them for their clinical judgment. Putting together the three data sources revealed a population inequity and an opportunity to improve both the individual patient's lives as well as the community's health. If we had not used multiple data sources to check the vitals in the sepsis program, these maternal sepsis cases could have been dismissed as outliers, rather than revealing a community-wide health disparity among Hispanic women.

This type of opportunity is why I strongly advocate for an integrated approach to data where metric data, case studies, and existing research are reviewed together. In data analytics, this process is called **data integration**. It is easy to slide into habit and rely on one data tool

---

3   The Centers for Medicare and Medicaid Services (2023). "Severe Sepsis Present." *Alphabetical Data Dictionary* (Version 5.14): 126. Retrieved on March 10, 2022, from https://qualitynet.cms.gov/inpatient/iqr.

or resource, but the best practice in data analytics is to integrate multiple sources to create a clear, big picture of the system and its problems.

Stepping Back

Author and retired Navy Seal Jocko Willink describes a tactical example of "stepping back" even when entering the danger zone under enemy fire. Without stepping back and detaching from the intensity of the task, he was unable to make decisions. But when he stepped back and focused on the bigger picture, he could see the problem clearly. He writes, by "stepping back off the firing line, and looking around—by detaching physically, even if only by a few inches, and, more important, detaching mentally from the problem at hand—I was able to see infinitely more than anyone else in my platoon."[4] This need to step back and see the big picture is why the three parts of a Vital Signs assessment are always considered together: Because data about the heart rate alone, with no knowledge of what is normal, and no report on whether or not there is chest pain would be useless – but the three together can reveal a more clear picture of the problem. When I need to get a better idea of what is really happening, I use a tool called the **Vital Signs Data Integration Tool**[5] to help me work through the different types of data, integrate the findings, and make decisions.

To reach a better understanding of data, however, I would like to share some key details about each of these three data sources. The following sections also include some Tech Tips on how to become comfortable using data, and an explanation of how these sources each contribute to the QI process. Last but not least, I will discuss hospital survey data, and how all of this information can be pulled together.

---

4   Willinck, J. (2020). First Platoon: Detach. *Leadership Strategy and Tactics*. St. Martin's Press.

5   Porter, G. (2022). "Vital Signs Data Integration Tool." PorterQI. https://porterqi.com/.

Existing Research

As soon as an issue is brought up as a potential problem, and before I talk to staff or look for clues about the origin and process of a problem, I try to start by looking at existing research. There are experts all over the world who look at common problems in healthcare and recommend evidence-based solutions for exactly the types of problems that our facilities experience. I try to take some time on each new problem to run a web search through professional organizations, or glance through online journals, and see if existing research has identified contributing factors and solutions to the problem. In the **Simple Tools** section, I share a list of quality organizations who publish research and curate position statements for best practices in healthcare, which is an excellent place to start looking for evidence-based practice recommendations as well as maintain current knowledge of best practices. As with any internet search, it helps to know which professional organizations will have the most current information, and the organizations listed in the **Simple Tools** chapter are part of an all-star cast for professional resources.

I have a confession to make: When I study existing research and keep an eye on measures that are being created by professional organizations, I have occasionally been able to make some useful predictions. It's like looking into the future to find out what will be expected of us next year. I discovered this by accident when the Severe Sepsis core measure was launched by CMS in 2015. My supervisor wanted to get a running start at implementing the core measure requirements, and there was a lot of pressure from the regional and corporate offices to perform well—but the guidelines were pushed back and would not be announced until it was uncomfortably close to when we would begin reporting compliance data to CMS. How would we build a program before we knew the expectations? I decided to look for the reason CMS had selected this measure above other issues in the first place and hoped to find a rationale in the process. I searched the research for information about

the sepsis bundle, which led me to The Sepsis Alliance[6] and a collaborative forum of clinicians in the same situation. The Sepsis Alliance
website, coupled with free CMS webinars, revealed a nice reference
list of journal articles. By reading the journal articles online, I found a
meta-analysis of multiple sepsis bundle studies and a complete list of the
treatments and assessments used in the original study protocol. So while
I lacked the actual guidance from CMS, I realized from the research
that recognition of sepsis was the first step to delivering rapid care and
increasing survival. I decided that I could start by educating staff on
early recognition while I waited for the detailed protocol to be revealed.
I was able to begin educating nursing staff about sepsis recognition
as "Wave 1" of our sepsis bundle project even though we did not yet
know what "Wave 2" would entail, simply because the existing research
emphasized staff recognition as the first, most important step to a
good sepsis program. The recognition of sepsis paved the way to deliver
the actual CMS bundle in "Wave 2" when it was announced, and our
nursing staff were already familiar with the need for early recognition
and urgent treatment—and our program was more successful because of
the early recognition training. This was an accidental discovery the first
time, but I quickly learned that checking existing research first could
keep me from floundering without a solid understanding of the problem
or the rationale for treatment.

Knowing the basis of research also helped tremendously when
physicians challenged the motivation of the Quality Department for
implementing the sepsis bundle: They wanted to know if this new
protocol was all about money and whether it really helped patient care?
I was able to share the meta-analysis I had found and provide evidence
for the work we were doing. No one wants to do extra work just to
improve numbers on paper, and I respect that our physicians cared
enough to ask hard questions about whether it would really make a
difference—they should question such things, and so should we. Now

---

6   The Sepsis Alliance (2022). About. Retrieved on March 14, 2022, from https://
www.sepsis.org/about/our-story/.

I start with existing research before I even look at facility-specific data, and certainly prior to designing any policies or protocols.

One final aspect of existing research that I cannot forget to mention is that it is essential to review existing policies at the facility. Sometimes a policy is out of date, sometimes there is no policy at all—but other times, there is a great policy that has just lost traction. A lot of delays can occur during the process of re-writing and changing policies, so it is important to thoroughly review what is already in place, identify the policy owner and talk to them, and be prepared to discuss the existing or retired policy when presenting any requested changes in committee meetings. I have found that it helps to bring a copy of the research support for any changes, and I try to speak personally with each policy owner or manager affected by the changes before bringing it up in a committee as a professional courtesy. When CMS creates a requirement, everyone understands that the change is not optional, but it is respectful to communicate about those changes at an individual level with leadership so that there are no surprises about how it will affect their team. These conversations can also provide advance warning of any barriers that could delay implementation, and it is also an opportunity to share the research about how these changes can improve patient care in their area. Of course, they may still not believe it will help patients until the real-time data comes in, and that is why the next section discusses how to use raw data effectively.

Raw Data

Raw Data typically comes from the electronic medical record and can be displayed and organized with several different tools and applications. Much of the information I use is displayed on giant spreadsheets that looked quite intimidating to me as a new QI professional. I had to invest time each week to develop skills in using spreadsheet applications like Excel™ to organize data and display it in a way that communicated effectively with others.

When I find a process or tool that I like, I write down the location of the tool in a notebook or document so that I can find it again. For example, if I wanted to remember how to save a document, I might write "Save: File > Save a copy > type the location" in my notes.

I also found reliable instructions for spreadsheet skills on the Microsoft Office™ Support website, which has video training for new users (https://support.microsoft.com). There are also training courses available through LinkedIn™ for several applications including Excel for a reasonable subscription fee (https://www.linkedin.com/learning). These courses are highly rated and can help professionals reach basic through advanced skills in data applications like Excel.

TECH TIP:

Some of the basic skills I frequently use include:

- **FAST FIND** a feature to locate key words in a data set (Ctrl + F)

- **ADD FILTER** button to use filters for sorting large columns and rows

- **COPY/PASTE AND SORTING** cells to display data clearly

- **FLASH FILL** to autofill a list similar to the input at the top of the list (Ctrl + E)

For someone who loves to learn new things, I can be a bit stubborn when it comes to new technology, resisting change and the constant flow of updates and "new looks" in the old applications I know. Every time my computer needs to update, I grumble, and I refused to get a smart phone until they had been around for several years. However, there is one aspect to keeping up with these tools that I would like to share: Fluent use of technology can save a tremendous amount of time on projects, and I like free time.

TECH TIP:

A couple of my favorite intermediate tools in Excel:

- **SUBTOTAL:** There are a few options in this function, but my favorite is the "count visible rows" feature, which allows me to sort a list with filters (hiding the patients I do not need to count) and count the visible rows only. For example, I might sort a list of psychiatric admissions by month and filter for restraint use, then use the SUBTOTAL tool to count the number of restraint incidents for the month.

- **PIVOT TABLE:** A pivot table is used to summarize data at a glance. It aggregates (pulls together) similar types of data into a clear display. I use pivot tables to summarize the pass rate for measures, or the number of employees meeting their hours each week.

- **XLOOKUP** AND **INDEX MATCH:** These tools are all used for large spreadsheets when I need to find a matching data point. For example, if you are looking through a list of patients who visited a specific unit and you want to find which ones also appear on a list of stroke patients, these tools would speed up that search by matching patient identifiers in both lists.

At one time, I needed to pull a list of over ten thousand patients each week, apply several formatting corrections, and remove duplicate entries for a mass upload. I spent four hours on the document the first time I worked on it, writing down the steps to make it clean and ready to publish in a personal process document for my notes. Then I looked for more efficient steps, and a colleague directed me to the "remove duplicates" button, along with several other tips and tricks in the spreadsheet application. I reduced the time spent on re-formatting each week to a half-hour session with only a few clicks thanks to those training resources, which meant I had three and a half hours added back into my "Metric Monday" weekly reporting. As my skills developed in using spreadsheets, I started learning how to use the features that helped me communicate visually, such as pivot tables and graphs, which display data in a more focused manner that is easier to understand. There were also formulas that helped me search large amounts of data for the few details I actually needed. These features are not immediately necessary, but they are convenient, and it is always a worthy professional goal to continue adding spreadsheet skills.

Data Sources

Since the patient chart and physician documentation are the locus of all healthcare data, it is important to learn how to pull patient lists by date range, diagnosis code, and discharge code. It came as a surprise to me that my familiarity with the live patient medical record did not necessarily prepare me for these tasks: While the bedside nurse is fluent in entering data, the review of data after discharge (retrospective) uses a different set of skills in a read-only format. I also discovered that my medical record user profile was completely different with "review" privileges instead of "live editing" privileges, which followed the security guidelines for my job description and permission to the "minimum necessary" access. Do not be afraid to ask for help from IT&S, or from a colleague in the administrative wing, to find and export these lists. It is possible that the ability to pull a specific patient list from the record may become part of a daily routine at some point and knowing how to ask for the list and move the data into a format that you can use will be a key skill.

Another source of raw data could be any paper form that departments still use, such as paper audits, which may or may not be scanned into the electronic record. Since these audits are both created and retired without much ado, it is good to reach out to local department leaders before writing forms from scratch for a new clinical project. There may be a repository of forms online, where the original template is available to print. In addition, hospital and department policies should be available in a library or index that is updated routinely, and the policy may indicate paper data sources, as well as the owner of the form and last official review. For example, the department manager of the psychiatric unit may have a paper restraint form to track incidents or audit documentation according to department policy. I also discovered that the operating room at my facility still used paper documentation due to sterile procedure requirements and logistics unique to that environment, so anesthesia reports were always on paper to be uploaded into the electronic medical record after the fact.

Some data tools aggregate (pull together) data from the medical record in a designed or pre-set format. There are so many tools for organizing and aggregating large amounts of data that it spawned a specialized field called **Data Analytics**. A lot of hospitals are devoting a significant amount of funding to build and maintain dashboards, for example, which are a single location to track data on problems determined to be a priority by leadership. Most of these dashboards allow you to export and download a range of raw data into a spreadsheet, and that raw data still comes from the patient's medical record and coding. Within the dashboard, the re-organized data may be displayed in percentages, ratios, or other metrics for quick comparison, but it is important to see how it is measured.

Beware Spoon-Fed Dashboards

Since the quality specialist is to be knowledgeable about the measures, I am cautious about taking the dashboard as my only reference, and I often need to explain to leadership why the dashboard shows the numbers it does or more often than not, explain information that does not make it to the dashboard. Since I am wary of spoon-fed data, I always look first for the "Export" icon on the dashboard, where I can find the original, raw data. If you cannot find an export icon, make it a priority with IT&S to insert that option in the next upgrade.

When I export to a spreadsheet, I can organize patient lists or other formats to reveal trends and contrasts that may not be visible in the summarized dashboard report. Using the original data, I may also find flaws in the sampling that could be improved in future iterations: It is important to note that the patient list being pulled into the dashboard may or may not match the patient lists that I am pulling locally—our methods may be different—and it is good to ask what the differences might be. Are the diagnosis codes for hemorrhagic stroke included or just ischemic? Does the dashboard include inpatient hospice patients? I found early on that I needed to make a habit of asking where the data came from and discuss what was included or excluded, and why. In QI, the details matter too much to assume that the lists are the same, and I have found that there can be dramatic differences. These differences and contrasts may be the answer to a problem my facility is facing and could help me capture a better picture of patient outcomes.

One example of frequently incongruent data that leads to mass chaos and confusion is the horrific use of percentages. I would caution anyone working with data to never, ever use a percentage without describing the total population it is based on, which is also called the sample size. Why were some numbers included or excluded? What are the raw numbers behind the percentage? For example, my regional supervisor called to discuss our sepsis mortality rates, and I honestly thought she was calling to congratulate us because only two people died of sepsis that month, compared to twelve the same month a year prior. However, my supervisor had noticed that our percentage of sepsis mortality was approaching 50%, and they had called to ask why our numbers were so bad. What happened?

Every percentage is only a reflection of the sample size: When only two people die in a population of four who become sick enough to be considered septic, there is a 50% rate of death. The year before, we had a pool of thirty people with sepsis and twelve of them died of septic shock. In real terms, twelve deaths are worse than two, and four people with severe sepsis is way, way better than thirty; fewer people were becoming severely ill with sepsis overall. We were saving lives. But when that life-saving work was displayed as a percentage without regard to the change in the total population of sepsis patients, it looked like nearly everyone was dying of sepsis at my hospital and the dashboard was bright red. Once we discussed the population numbers, and the sepsis program in general, my regional supervisor decided that we were doing a great job and started a new project to review the severity of illness among sepsis patients in the region.

The issue of population and sample size is an important one: We are trying to help patients get better and go home, which means we are really measuring against perfection—a high standard to be sure, but not too high when it affects real human beings. If we measure against a low standard—a population we know we'll look good against—we may "standardize" ill health, disparities, or poor outcomes, reinforcing the problem rather than improving it.

The Mortality Index

This predicament of sampling data is one of the reasons why the Mortality Index was created. With a Mortality Index, patients could be compared to similar populations by diagnosis and risk (an equal standard). There are many "really sick patients" in hospitals but being sick should not necessarily lead to death. When we study mortality, we especially want to know if a death was likely to happen anyway, or if the quality of care affected the outcome in some way. The Mortality Index is one way to determine if quality of care needs to be investigated when a mortality occurs; it considers whether a death was expected and includes a risk adjustment for underlying health issues and the likelihood of a terminal outcome. Specifically, the Mortality Index is a ratio of deaths actually Observed against the number of deaths Expected for the age (O/E) and risk of the population. A perfect match between actual deaths and expected deaths would be an index score of 1, and a ratio of greater than 1 is considered an excessive mortality score. For example, a Mortality Index ratio for someone whose cause of death was a stroke might be 1.17 if the patient had no other problems—meaning observed deaths were greater than expected and the patient was not expected to die. However, the Mortality Index ratio might be 0.98 if the stroke patient also had blood pressure problems, diabetes, kidney disease, and a recent terminal lung cancer diagnosis to indicate the death was expected.

By measuring this way, hospitals are not penalized when they treat "really sick patients" with deadly illnesses because the population and context is weighed against the occurrences of death. When the Mortality Index ratio is greater than one, hospitals should review mortality cases individually and look for reasons the mortalities occurred, looking for any adjustments and opportunities to improve patient care (see Mortality Review in the "Simple Tools" section of Chapter Four for more details).

In summary, data analysis is not just a place for pencil pushers and accountants. In the world of Healthcare QI, it can and should be used to save patient lives and improve their quality of care. To do that, the QI professional should be aware of where a metric comes from, how and why it was selected, and what was excluded. It is also helpful to remember that the display tools (tables, graphs, etc.) are just that—they are tools to help us see the story within the available data, but they are not the data itself. The real information is often in the giant spreadsheets and becoming comfortable with searching and navigating large data sets is an essential skill to build and maintain in any QI role.

But what happens if the existing research and the raw data do not answer the question or effectively explain the problem? The next type of data is the one that makes me feel most like an old-fashioned detective with the Sherlock Holmes hat and a magnifying glass: subjective interviews, patient tracers, and case studies—with just a dash of the mysterious plot twists that even Agatha Christie might appreciate.

Subjective Studies

Another way to look at patient care at a more personal, qualitative level is through the lens of subjective tracers and case studies. The focus of this type of data is to tell the story of an event so that we can learn about it — like the obstetric sepsis alerts that were presented at the beginning of this chapter; the story of the patient going through septic shock showed that there was a real need for sepsis alerts in the obstetrics department. Subjective studies help QI professionals remember the human side behind all the numbers and often reveal solutions that would not be found in raw data alone.

The first type of subjective study is called a "tracer,"[7] and it is a tool that Joint Commission (TJC) uses frequently when they conduct a facility survey for certification. A "tracer" is when they trace a patient chart from the point of entry to the point of discharge and evaluate safety throughout the encounter. Tracers create a kind of case study by documenting a patient's story throughout their visit, and I have found that creating similar case studies that follow patients through multiple units can be extremely helpful in implementing new protocols and programs for QI, especially if they may be affected by transfers or unit-specific differences. Tracers are great for looking at a process.

The second type of subjective study we'll discuss is a case study, which can be as simple as a walk through the patient experience asking "Why?" and taking notes on anything unusual or interesting. A case study may include staff or management interviews about the case to ask for clarification. To create a focused case study, I usually review critical test results and provider notes, and write a descriptive sentence about each day of the stay until the patient expired or discharged. I then summarize those findings on a table where I pull relevant information such as code status, fluid administration, and discharge status, along with a brief description of the patient's encounter. This data gave me a subjective bird's eye view of the patient's progress and care. Where tracers are focused on the process and flow of a patient's care, case studies are more thematic and can look at the details of a diagnosis or the influence of a particular quality program.

Case studies can also be used to provide a specific example of what might be typical for a population or as an educational example. Going back to the sepsis example, many Emergency Department (ED) physi-

---

7   The Joint Commission (2022). Tracer methodology. Retrieved March 15, 2022, from https://www.jointcommission.org/resources/news-and-multimedia/fact-sheets/facts-about-tracer-methodology/.

cians across the nation expressed concern in the sepsis forums about complying with the sepsis fluid bolus required by CMS. Locally, we investigated the outcome of our sepsis patients, but the ED physicians were not permitted by HIPAA to see whether sepsis patients survived after transferring to the ICU with or without fluid. Since they could see patients experience fluid overload immediately in the ED, they were opposed to giving fluid. Due to HIPAA, no one could just tell the ED physicians that the patients are better because of the bolus, but as a QI professional, I could review the sepsis cases and de-identify the patient charts. So we gathered real-life data as anonymous case studies, demonstrating survival compared to fluid bolus compliance, and we could then have a robust discussion about the importance of the fluid bolus for long-term survival. Even though fluid overload was rare and death from sepsis was common, it was natural to worry about the immediate risk of fluid overload because that was what they saw during the time they cared for the patient. Without a case study, they could not see the improved outcome with fluid, or the increased risk of not receiving fluid.

The fluid discussion led to another important conversation about what to do when a patient with comorbidities wanted "everything done" and declined Comfort Measures Only (CMO). Should they give the fluid? Would the patient want to be intubated? This discussion would improve patient care and highlight the need to discuss the patient's goals of care early in the encounter rather than later. Without the case study examples, the ED physicians would have remained distrustful of the fluid recommendations, but with a case study it becomes easier to talk about why the fluid was recommended with such broad applications, and how to apply the protocol without causing harm or failing to obtain the patient's wishes before the need for resuscitation.

Subjective System Studies

Case studies or tracers can also be conducted on a system rather than an individual. This approach can be useful when there is potential for a community or population-based issue, or maybe a trend on a particular unit. My colleague, the stroke coordinator, found that the number of stroke alerts quadrupled during winter months and decided to conduct an informal tracer on the stroke unit during that timeframe: The stroke coordinator was visiting each stroke patient to personalize their stroke education, and he began to ask questions about what brought them to the area and how did they notice their stroke symptoms, recording those findings in his notes. This tracer revealed an increase in elderly, long-term visitors during the winter due to the warm, southern climate. This seasonal population change was directly correlated to the increase in our stroke alerts during winter months, as well as an increase in mortality. Based on this data, we implemented education programs for stroke prevention and recognition that targeted community centers for elderly winter visitors and adapted our education program to ensure that every patient received personalized stroke education.

As a tool for research, case studies do not include judgement about actions taken, but should report facts that would be important to the patient in something that resembles a story or narrative format. It is about telling the patient story and identifying opportunities in greater detail than just numbers, and it allows for the implications of a problem to be reviewed and discussed in a professional manner.

Survey Data & Peer Review

I learned in school that it helps to have someone check my work before I submit embarrassing spelling errors about "Bare Activity in the Forest" to the teacher. In college, I learned that peer review is a method of verifying data and ensuring that research studies meet the standards of the profession. In a lot of ways, hospital surveys are like a peer review for our quality and safety programs: Hospitals pay organizations like

The Joint Commission (TJC)[8] and Det Norske Veritas (DNV)[9] to visit their facility and conduct a live audit, or "survey," of patient quality and safety. The purpose of the survey is to ensure that the facility is applying best practices and meeting the standards of the industry. Facilities that pass their survey obtain accreditation from the organization, which can be advertised to the public as a sign of diligence to the standards of healthcare quality and safety. The accreditation lasts for a specific period of time called a "survey cycle" and must be renewed within that timeframe to maintain the accreditation.

During a survey, experts from the accrediting organization choose a selection of patients representing high-risk categories that are sampled and a patient tracer is conducted. Individual units are audited, and staff may be interviewed for their knowledge of specific standards, infection control techniques, medication management, and other key topics in quality and safety. When fault is found in the existing process, it may be called a Requirement For Improvement (RFI), where the facility would then need to demonstrate that they have made the necessary changes to receive accreditation for the following survey cycle. These RFIs may also be scored on a risk matrix to indicate the frequency of the incident against the potential harm it could cause.

The standards of care examined in these hospital survey audits evolve based on risks identified in healthcare quality and safety outcomes data. In the "Brief History" section of Chapter One, I mentioned Deming's approach to manufacturing outcomes and the search for any variation from the expected outcome. This emphasis on patient outcomes is still a driving force in Healthcare QI, where patient harm and unexpected deaths continue to determine which QI topics will take priority each year.

While each facility is responsible for training staff on best practices,

8   The Joint Commission (2022). Who We Are. Retrieved on Aug. 10, 2022, from https://www.jointcommission.org/who-we-are/facts-about-the-joint-commission/.

9   Det Norske Veritas (2022). Hospital Accreditation. Retrieved on Aug. 10, 2022, from https://www.dnv.com/services/hospital-accreditation-7516/.

as well as monitoring for compliance, some facilities that are affiliated with a larger healthcare system may have a regional or corporate auditing team visit and conduct a "mock survey" to test the facility on their survey readiness. These mock surveys are often intentionally more rigorous than the official ones, as they are testing the preparedness of the hospital team. Basically, a mock survey is like taking a test preparation course where potential weaknesses are reviewed, and plans are made to get ready for the official test and ensure a passing score.

During a survey, key members from the leadership team walk with the auditors as they ask questions, review current medical records, and interview staff. Several members of the quality and patient safety team are typically invited to join the survey team as note-takers and representatives, ensuring that no advisory comments will be missed. Following the survey, a complete review of findings will be conducted by the auditors, and further questions may be asked about RFIs and any required changes. After the survey, a decision about accreditation is made by the auditing team.

When it is time for renewal, a timeframe is noted when the surveyors may return unannounced and begin their audit. In the meantime, the data from an RFI will require an action plan by the facility to demonstrate the required changes were made. Each action plan will need to be based on the RFI findings, and any new policies or measurements will need to be available at the time of the next survey. For example, this can be as simple as an audit tool to ensure that all food stored in staff refrigerators is labeled appropriately, or it may involve creating a new policy for safe storage of surgical implants, or facility-wide training and audits on the safe use of physical restraints for patients with a high injury risk. If the accreditation is program-specific, such as a stroke certification survey, the data to support program progress will need to be up-to-date and readily available.

Regardless of the presence or lack of an RFI, all survey data will play an important role in decision-making and prioritization of projects for the QI professional because survey data is focused on the outcomes that matter most to patients.

Putting It All Together

To summarize, how would I put these data sources together to make sense of a problem? In the most basic terms, I would start with existing research from respected organizations and journals, then pull patient data by the code or population of interest, and finally, do a case study on some of the outliers, patients who died, or cases that were unusual. If I found a unique problem (like obstetric sepsis), I would start over and look for existing research on the new, focused problem.

Finally, if the data becomes overwhelming, it is important to remember what matters to all of our patients. If I ask the patient what their priority is, the answer is clear: The patient wants to walk out of the hospital and go home. No one wants to stay in the hospital, and most people (even the terminally ill) do not wish to die in the hospital given the choice.[10] So when I am dealing with massive amounts of data, I sometimes ask, "What will help the patient discharge home safely?" The answer helps me filter through the data and find what matters most to our patients. The unchanging nature of the fact that all our patients want to leave the hospital alive and, if it is within our power, in better condition than they arrived can help guide our decisions in healthcare data analytics, as any exception to these patients' goals is truly an opportunity for improvement.

10   Gomes, B.; Calanzani, N.; Koffman, J.; and Higginson, I.J. (Oct. 9, 2015). Is dying in hospital better than home in incurable cancer and what factors influence this? A population-based study. *BMC Medicine* (13): 235.

Chapter 3
Project Management

Often times when we hear the term "project management," we think of gurus in formal wear standing in front of flow charts on a screen, shuffling boxes around like Tom Cruise in *Minority Report*—and since Cruise plays a detective in that movie, there's a part of me that really resonates with that metaphor. But now that I have been part of project-management teams, I know "project management" includes way more scientific method than Sherlockian intuition.

The first time someone told me about the scientific method, I was deeply disappointed. I really thought I was going to learn how to use a Bunsen burner to make candles, start an earthquake with a paperclip, or learn something else really cool. But the scientific method is so simple: Ask a question, try something, check back to see what happened. For example, I was a scientist when my four-year-old self asked, "Would rubbing banana all over my face be the same as wearing make-up like my mom?" It did not, but at least I learned the answer to my question.

The Nursing Process

Later in life, I learned that the the Nursing Process was like the scientific method of professional nursing. The Nursing Process[1] is essential to helping nurses deliver holistic, patient-centered care. Nurses need an evidence-based rationale for patient interventions then they determine the patient needs, deliver care, and check back to see what happened. As a nurse moving from a bedside position into an administrative role, I was delighted, however, when I found out that Quality Improvement

---

1   Potter, P. A., & Perry, A. G., et al (2004). Nursing Assessment. *Fundamentals of Nursing* (6th ed.): 279. Mosby.

(QI) principles are strikingly similar to both the scientific method and the Nursing Process, except they are applied to systems rather than an experiment or an individual patient.

Before we dive into the details of the Nursing Process and how it applies to QI projects, let's consider what nursing and QI already share: The purpose of both bedside nursing and QI is to advocate and care for patients holistically. At the bedside, sometimes there were small problems that were a big deal to patients—like a missing cell phone that was a lifeline between an elderly patient and their family, or missing glasses that kept a patient from being able to sign their surgical consent and could result in treatment delays. In nursing, we worked hard to advocate for our patients and solve their problems, digging through the trash and looking under furniture for the missing item. In QI, we look for the source of those problems and try to fix the process or system that caused it to happen in the first place; every patient is our patient. We look for the reason those items were lost, but the reason we look is because it matters to the patient. One of the sections below is about identifying the problem, and this patient-centered approach will come up again, because QI professionals are not about pushing paper. We are all about helping the patient, and we use a process to ensure that we have found the right problem at the right time and that our solution really works.

The scientific method, the nursing process, and all of the QI processes, have the same general structure with small differences in depth and attention:

1. Ask a question

2. State the problem

3. Gather evidence and measurements

4. Change something

5. Study what happened after the change

In QI, the question is the same: How can we improve the quality of patient care?

For nurses, gathering evidence means assessing a patient and taking their history then collaborating with the healthcare team to deliver relevant interventions. In QI project management, the process is similar, but the evidence comes from larger sources. I have found that it helps to see the Nursing Process and QI methods side-by-side to understand the process of QI project management. I have included a breakdown of a generic improvement process next to the nursing process, but we will also go into more detail later in this chapter:

TABLE 3.1 FEATURED TOOL: QUALITY IMPROVEMENT PROCESS	
NURSING PROCESS	**QUALITY IMPROVEMENT PROCESS**
Assessment	Look for problems by pulling large amounts of patient data and searching for poor results
Diagnosis	Identify a priority problem
Planning	Develop tracking documents
Implementation	Start making changes
Evaluation	Decide whether the planned change solved the initial problem, repeat as necessary

Basically, the "patient" for a QI professional is the hospital system with all the people, processes, and projects that exist because they matter to real patients. In the following sections, I will walk through some examples and observations about applying the Nursing Process step-by-step to improve quality at a hospital.

Assessment: Look for Problems

The first step in the process is to find out how the system is doing with an assessment. The assessment stage of the process is just like the Nursing Admission Assessment. The bedside nurse cannot assume anything, and every aspect of the patient's physical condition and history must be assessed before a problem can be identified or a diagnosis made. In a hospital system, the quality professional cannot assume anything and must perform an assessment to obtain an overview of the system's health. Here are some basic questions to ask during the assessment:

- What are the worst results for patients right now?
  - o Example: Unexpected deaths in mortality review, hospital-acquired conditions, patient harm, delays in care, below threshold quality scores

- What are patients and employees saying right now about quality of care?
  - o Example: HCAHPS survey results, staff interviews, near-miss event reporting, staff participation in committees and councils

- What is the top priority of hospital leadership right now, and why?
  - o Example: Public reporting, hospital survey results, staffing expenses and overtime, supply shortages

- What matters most to medical staff, and why?
  - o Example: Computerized physician order entry, barriers to scheduling an operating suite, consistency of nursing care, independence of practice, barriers to maintaining privileges and credentialing

- What problems are CMS and TJC focusing on this year?
  - o Example: Alarm fatigue, stroke management, anticoagulant monitoring, patient falls with injury

These questions are like the patient history. As a nurse, I knew that I could not care for every diagnosis and symptom that a patient might have, but when I chose a priority nursing diagnosis, I needed to know the whole picture before I could consider what action to take. If I discovered that my pneumonia patient had diabetes, I may or may not make a nursing plan for comprehensive diabetes care, but I would certainly consider that diabetes may affect the patient's recovery from the infection causing the pneumonia as I planned their care. Likewise, the usage rates of computerized physician order entry (CPOE) among medical staff may not be at the top of the facility's priority list, but it could influence priority projects like the certification of the stroke program. The broad questions listed above will elicit a massive amount of information, but the next step will be setting priorities for the most severe problems among that broad array of issues (which we will discuss shortly).

When performing this QI assessment, it is also important to keep the hospital administration's goals in the forefront. The leadership team members each have access to a big picture that the QI professional may not see, and invested support from administration and medical staff is critical to the success of any QI project, so it is a good idea to attend administrative meetings to be aware of what is important to the leadership team and be ready to answer questions about quality projects. In contrast, it is extremely difficult to improve a problem if administration is not involved and invested because each project requires research, education, and staff hours that either help or hurt the bottom line of hospital finances, and they are gatekeepers to these resources. With a healthy partnership, however, administrative support can help shift funding and incentives to promote projects that QI professionals believe will make a significant positive impact, and the QI professional can design a project that is useful to the administrative goals, incorporating their input on cost, staffing, and resource management.

After gathering a broad history with the questions above, those questions can be used to create a list of project opportunities or problems. Those projects can be ranked in a problem-specific assessment to further organize the problems, looking for details about specific problems so that decisions can be made about priorities, goals, and resources. I like to use a very rough adaptation of the Failure Modes and Effects Analysis (FMEA) tool to assess which problems have the greatest scope of impact.

FEATURED TOOL: FMEA

The FMEA tool was created by the military to identify all the ways a project could fail.[2] It lists out categories of areas where failure could occur, and then cascades through those problems, imagining failure at every step. Then these failures are rated by levels of severity. The purpose is to find solutions to major issues before the failure actually happens, but it also gives a guideline about which failures would be the most urgent and severe. So an FMEA basically scores the most important problems in a complex process. While the concept of scoring a problem by how much it affects patients is not difficult to understand, the FMEA form itself is quite a headache. So let's take a look at a simplified version:

Instructions: Rank each category with a score of **Low (1), Moderate (2), or High (3)**.

- What is the severity of the problem? This assessment asks for a rank to identify the risk of harm associated with a problem. Will it cause certain death or catastrophe? A potential lawsuit? A shortage of pencils?

- How often does this problem occur? Also called the frequency, this assessment tries to count the number of incidents over a specific amount of time. Does the problem happen every week, or is it a rare occurrence?

- How easy is it to track and measure the problem? This assessment looks at the constraints and feasibility of monitoring progress. When the problem occurs, is it easy

---

2   Tague, Nancy (2005). *The Quality Toolbox* (2nd edition). ASQ Quality Press.

to identify? Is there a report available for this problem? For instance, sepsis is hard to identify, but septic shock is obvious; patient fall risk is hard to guess, but when someone falls, it is a clear problem.

Once the problems are scored, tally the scores, and set aside the ones that have the highest scores: These are problems that are having a serious effect on a lot of patients and can be feasibly improved.

From this new list of severe problems affecting lots of patients, is there a way to filter them down to something as simple as the ABCs of Resuscitation (Airway, Breathing, and Circulation) to find the most important QI problem at a facility?

Yes, there is! And I will share it in the next section about identifying the priority problem.

Diagnosis: Identify a Priority Problem

After the facility-wide assessment and problem-ranking, the list of high-impact problems is likely still too large and broad to make decisions about specific projects. Rather, the high-impact problem list should be used to set project priorities based on criteria that matters most to patients. The rationale is not just that patients are the customer, but that a good outcome for patients in one area (fewer falls) tends to come back as a good outcome in other areas (fewer readmissions, decreased cost, and higher patient satisfaction scores). The greatest positive effect for a healthcare facility is found by focusing on the greatest positive outcomes for patients.

Most people in healthcare would not argue against a patient-as-priority philosophy, but how do we identify what matters to patients? It's not like patients greet their doctors with questions about pressure-ulcer rates, but we all know that nobody wants a wound on their back. So how do we advocate for patients without just speaking over them?

FEATURED TOOL: THE ABCS (ACUTE, BIG, COSTLY)

Patient priorities can be organized by the ABCs of Acute, Big, and Costly to identify the problems that would be most concerning to the patient:

A: Acute: How much harm comes from this problem?

Using Deming's model of focusing on outcomes and looking for variations from the expected outcome, I always come back to the reality that patients do not want to die or be harmed during their encounter: If there is an issue that is causing excess mortality or patient harm, that is the issue that should take priority: It is a variance from the expected norm. If there were any medical errors or evidence of negligence, then leadership, risk management, and patient safety will need to be involved as well.

B: Big: How widespread is this problem?

Problems are more severe if they represent a trend or a habit rather than an isolated incident. Asking how many patients are affected or whether the problem is present in more than one location can identify whether a staff write-up will solve the problem, or whether an entire process needs to change.

C: Costly: Is the problem expensive?

If the problem results in repeated expenses, loss of life, or heavy litigation, it is an expensive problem. Likewise, if the problem results in a reduction in the performance payment rate from Medicare, it can be unbelievably costly (see Abstraction and Public Reporting chapter for more details).

Getting the Problem Wrong

I'm going to be brutally honest: Identifying the problem is usually the part of the process that goes wrong. I typically want to jump in and start solving problems, and when I see a lot of problems building up, it seems like a pointless redundancy to sit around talking about which problem we should pick from the vast supply of available issues. Talk about bureaucracy, right? We just need to get started and do something! However, experience has taught me not to rush this step.

Why is it so difficult to identify the priority problem? Most of us know what the elephant in the room is, right?

WRONG.

Identifying the problem is the most challenging part of the QI process. Psychologists have reported a phenomenon called inattentional blindness where tasks requiring focus "can act like a set of blinders." because our brains use selective attention to focus on relevant stimuli and dismiss irrelevant stimuli.[3] This selective attention helps us solve complex problems, but it also helps magicians fool our minds with illusions and distraction.[4]

In a clinical example, one study asked 24 radiologists to perform a routine lung nodule detection task. There was just one catch: An image of a gorilla was placed in an upper lobe of the lung scans. Did the radiologists laugh and report that there was a picture of a gorilla waving at them in the upper lobes? On the contrary, 83% of the radiologists in the study did not even mention the waving gorilla. They were so focused on the task of detecting lung nodules that they missed the big picture. Most of the time, we can't even see the elephant in the room, much less address it.

Inattentional blindness is how we miss entire population health

3   Drew, T.; Yo, M.; Wolfe, J. (Sept. 2013). The invisible gorilla strikes again: Sustained inattentional blindness in expert observers. *Psychol Sci* (9): 1848-53.

4   Lehrer, J. (Aug. 2021). The Magic Gasp. *Mystery: A Seduction, A Strategy, A Solution*. Simon & Schuster.

issues, like the obstetric sepsis example in the **Data Analysis** chapter. It is why we should never trust ourselves when we think we know exactly what to do about a problem, and it is why we work so hard to identify the root of a problem after considering every aspect of the data. Identifying the priority problem will help identify a real solution, rather than running around wildly to fix random problems that would just happen again. Without a plan, our solutions would look like someone putting sunblock on a sunburn and thinking no harm will come from going back to sit on the beach all day. Clearly, the sunburn would only get worse from ongoing ultraviolet damage because sunblock was never meant to be used as a burn-healer, but as a safeguard to prevent burns from happening. We must focus our efforts and find the priority problem in the data if we want to use our resources effectively and see lasting success.

To understand what it looks like to find a priority problem and design a project around it, I've provided an example situation that I will walk through in detail throughout this chapter, illustrating how each step applies to the problem.

EXAMPLE PROBLEM:

Problem: Patient survey scores are below threshold and several patients commented that they lost their belongings after a procedure, which affected their HCAHPS satisfaction scores.

Situation: Hospital leadership states that they would like to see improved HCAHPS scores become a priority. Although no one will die if belongings go missing (it is not an "acute" problem), the public reporting of low HCAHPS scores that specifically mention lost belongings, combined with the cost of replacing missing items (it is "costly"), has made this problem a priority for leadership. It is also a pervasive problem that affects a significant number of patients ("big"). While the problem of lost patient belongings would not override a series of mysterious, unexpected deaths on the priority problem list, it can easily take second place as a moderate-level priority due to low cost and broad scope.

Evidence: Raw data from the HCAHPS surveys showed that most patient complaints reported that belongings were lost after a procedure.

Working Problem Statement: The post anesthesia care unit (PACU) is the origin of the problem. PACU staff are likely distracted and are inattentive to patient belongings.

Possible Intervention: A post-op checklist that audits patient belongings could improve staff attention to the issue.

Question: Is this the priority problem? Is there any other data that should be gathered?

At this point, raw survey data was reviewed, but is there a review of existing research that can be useful? There may not be a lot of existing research on the subject of patient belongings beyond security issues and mitigation of lawsuits, but there should be an existing policy at the facility. The patient belongings policy states that patients will be offered use of the hospital safe for their valuables and that any other belongings should be given to their family or a caregiver, but clearly, something is not working with this process; otherwise, the HCAHPS surveys would be more positive.

What about subjective interviews? We can ask the manager about the normal process for stowing belongings for operative patients. Also, this is a great time for us to put on a detective's hat, grab a clipboard and head over to PACU to look for clues: We can talk to the nurses and ask them why they think the items were lost. After sleuthing around the PACU, we find that not all patients had family with them, so belongings could not be given to a family member. Putting all belongings in the hospital safe was not happening because patients did not want to surrender critical items like reading glasses, cell phones, and dentures; they wanted them to be available as soon as they got out of surgery. Further, the entire operative wing of the hospital is not stocked with patient belonging bags, so there was no way to send items with the patient safely.

Let's pause and see what we have so far:

Situation: Patient survey scores are below threshold, and several patients commented that they lost their belongings after a procedure, which affected their HCAHPS satisfaction scores.

Evidence:

- Raw data from the HCAHPS surveys showed that nearly all patient complaints reported that belongings were lost after a procedure.

- The existing policy was to ask family to hold belongings or put them in the safe.

- Interviews with staff revealed that many patients want to keep their cell phone, glasses, and dentures with them, but patient belonging bags are not stocked in the operating wing.

Working Problem Statement: PACU staff have no safe place to put patient belongings.

Question: Is this the root cause of the problem? Why did this problem occur?

Another technique in identifying the priority problem is to continue asking "Why?" until there is no other answer to give. When we asked, "Why are the PACU nurses losing patient belongings?" we found out that there is no safe place to put them. Can we still ask why? "Why is there no safe place to put patient belongings?" At this point, we might begin to get curious about the ordering system. When we ask about the process of ordering patient belonging bags, the manager informs us that there is no way to order them because they are not on the floor's order forms. Why?

Later, in a discussion with the supply chain manager, we find that the belonging bags were never added to PACU's ordering forms because of the previously discovered policy stating that operative patients would give their belongings to family or place them in the hospital safe. They do not need belongings bags because their belongings are supposed to be handed off to others, not stay with the patients. So the question, "Why is there no safe place to put these items?" was answered with the barrier to ordering belonging bags, and "Why can't bags be ordered?" was answered with a missing line on a supply chain form, which resulted from the policy we discovered during our earliest research, which does not reflect patient preference and department habit.

Now, our evidence chain looks like this:

Evidence:

- Raw data from the HCAHPS surveys showed that nearly all patient complaints reported that belongings were lost after a procedure.

- The existing policy was to ask family to hold belongings.

- Interviews revealed that many patients want to keep their cell phone, glasses, and dentures with them, but patient belonging bags are not stocked in the operating wing.

- The PACU manager stated that there is no way to order patient belonging bags for PACU to use because the supply form is based on department policy.

- The department policy on patient belongings is not updated to reflect patient preference and department procedures.

We have certainly come a long way from identifying staff distraction as the source of the problem (and probably saved a bunch of people from getting write-ups). We are beginning to form an evidence-based diagnosis for our priority problem. Having what seems to be a full picture, there are a number of feasible opportunities in this case, including updating the lacking policy and adding a line item for belongings bags on the order form. Presenting the problem to administrators offers an easy buy-in because there is a low-cost solution that will improve scores and outcomes. Of course, to truly know if the priority problem was identified, we would need to measure whether these changes decreased the incidence of missing belongings, and this data will not be available until the end of the project. But even without this ideal resolution, the PACU staff and management are already happy to discover process problems with potential solutions and staff morality improves.

Experts in quality are always saying that we should avoid assigning blame to staff for problems and should instead try to find the non-human part of the process that made it possible for the problem to exist in the first place. Looking at a process requires diligence to discover the first problem that set all the other ones in motion. The priority problem in our example is about updating policy to reflect reality, and improving the availability of belonging bags because those problems rank higher than measuring how many PACU nurses complete an audit: These process errors address a root cause, not just a symptom of the root cause. Truly, these investigations are a big part of the "detective work" that I love so much. Every problem is a mystery until all the clues are gathered, witnesses interviewed, and the source of the problem is identified. My favorite problems are the ones with red herrings that distract me and a twist in the plot near the end of the analysis.

I will admit that sometimes when I dig into a problem that I have suspected was a systemic problem, I find it is not as big of an issue as I suspected, and I need to make a choice: Maybe it is a signal to look at the data in a new way, or it may be a personal hang-up that is not really a priority for patient care. It is okay to let things go if they are not the priority today. For those issues, I like to keep a list of things that are low priority, and if I catch up on my scheduled work, I always have something to brainstorm and investigate (that did actually happen once).

Once a priority problem is identified, it is time to choose a method for measuring improvements or changes that will be made. How will we know if our changes are solving the problem? That step will require some planning.

FEATURED TOOL: UTOPIAN HOSPITAL

If I get stuck, there is one other tool that I like to pull out: Envision what excellent patient care would look like and work backwards from that vision. I know that sounds incredibly silly to many people, but it is so motivating to picture the way things could be for our own communities, and it can help us focus on the pursuit of solutions rather than chasing problems in a reactive manner.

Working backwards from an ideal is also a great way to start thinking about how to measure a problem; it is common to lean on a burdensome audit when working forwards from the problem itself, but it may well be easier to innovate from the ideal. Usually, as soon as the audit goes away, the problems it solved slowly begin to return. In an ideal situation, staff will want to complete the tasks we were auditing because they want to help their patients, and for the most part, they do these things without thinking. It's second nature.

How did we get to that cultural change?

These brainstorming sessions can help identify a feasible way to track change, reduce paperwork, and improve patient care.

Planning: Measure the Problem

After spending most of our day identifying the problem, it is finally time to look for ways to measure the problem and plan for how it might change.

PROBLEM SUMMARY: Hospital leadership set a priority for improving HCAHPS scores because the patient belongings problem was Big and Costly. Since it is affordable to implement, they ask that the project occur immediately, which is feasible since the proposed interventions require very little expense or time. Planning begins for implementation of this moderate-level priority.

PROPOSED INTERVENTIONS INCLUDE:

1) Updating the policy for keeping patient belongings safe during procedures.

2) Adding patient belonging bags to the supply chain par-stock form.

3) Informing staff of the changes to the patient belongings policy in the next staff huddle.

One measurement choice that must be made is whether we will measure the occurrence of the problem or the compliance rate of the solution. It will be easy to check-off our paperwork to-do list and say that we measured something, but simply making changes to paperwork will not show whether belongings are safe or if patients are happier with their care: We need information about the desired patient outcome and not just the project outcome. For example, most treatment protocols would measure if the solution was delivered on time (compliance), but for most error reduction problems, we usually want to measure the problem's occurrence. In this case, if we measure the occurrence of the problem, we will find out if the problem is still happening, but if we measure compliance with the solution, we will likely need to create a new real-time performance audit on safe belongings—something we were hoping to avoid.

To better illustrate this decision, imagine a manager asking an employee to clean the office. The employee determines that they will need cleaning supplies to fulfill this request, so cleaning supplies are moved into the office. Now imagine that the employee checks cleaning off their list and reports to the manager that the job is done. It was not wrong to put cleaning supplies in the office—it was a necessary step, and it was not wrong to create a checklist—that is a helpful reminder. But at the end of the day, the manager will have to return to the original problem statement and see if the office is clean or dirty. The measurement then is not the whether there was an action or the whether the documentation is complete; the measurement is the real-world effect of those implementations. Whenever action is taken, it is important to return to the problem statement and ask, "Is the problem resolved? If not, what's missing?" Selecting whether we will measure how much the problem is occurring or how effectively the solution is getting done is about finding the best way to ask this question.

In our belongings case, it is probably more effective to measure if the problem is still occurring: We want to know if these changes will improve HCAHPS scores for operative patients, and it would be nice to track the incidence of lost belongings due to their cost. We discover that it's difficult to obtain real-time tracking of lost items, although we can at least track the expense of replacing those items after discharge. We could give a focused discharge survey about satisfaction with keeping patient belongings safe in the surgical department so that we can measure in real time, but there are no baseline discharge surveys for comparison. Perhaps the best option would be to wait for HCAHPS scores to show an increase in satisfaction and compare it to the baseline survey data.

The measurement stage can be a time when the problem becomes more focused as we begin to discuss it with the departments who are affected, pull more specific data, and draft staff education about the project. Sometimes the measurement tool is pre-selected because it is a national or corporate metric. Other times, the goal is based on a repeatable measurement of the current problem.

Starting with the problem statement, the evidence gathered in the initial assessment may reveal opportunities for measurement: Is it possible to count the number of times the problem occurs in a day, week, or month? Does the problem always occur at a certain location? Measurement can occur at any time during the patient's experience: A problem could be measured before, during, or after an event, for example. Sometimes we measure outcomes at discharge, or sometimes it is better to identify at-risk patients early in their stay and tag them for closer monitoring. For example, research showed that early identification and treatment was crucial for managing acute stroke.[5] Since any delay in treatment could increase the risk of disability, early identification and treatment upon arrival would be necessary to prevent patient harm. However, in the case of missing items, the problem is not life-threatening, and there is plenty of time to measure outcomes during or after discharge.

When examining raw data about patients currently affected by the problem, otherwise known as the sample for the problem in the study, it's not always easy to figure out how to find that population in the system. There may be cross-over diagnosis codes, overlapping processes, and other factors that can make it difficult to clearly define. It may help to ask which group or sample would most clearly reveal the problem you are studying and which groups could be affected by other problems or variables. Select the simplest, most clearly defined sample that you can find so that it does not confuse the measurement of the solution. For the patient belongings project, this might include a daily census of procedures, or patients discharging from the surgical ward, or the next HCAHPS report; the sample needs to be large enough to show whether the process is working. As another example, most stroke patients came to the Emergency Department and triggered a stroke alert that would be clearly documented, so stroke alert notifications in the ED would be a manageable sample to study. I still like to do a pilot of my own where I try the measurement tool and see if it actually "captures" patients correctly. If not, I would return to the problem statement and see what other characteristics or demographics I could try to pull into a sample or spreadsheet for measurement.

In many ways, after all the tedious work with spreadsheets and committees, it is a relief to finally talk about measuring the goal. I like getting to ask more encouraging questions, like "At what point would these changes make a real, tangible difference for patients?" That

---

5   Gotz, T., Gerloff, C. (2015). Treatment Concepts for Wake-Up Stroke and Stroke With Unknown Time of Symptom Onset. *Stroke, 2015* (46), 2707-2713. https://doi. org/10.1161/STROKEAHA.115.009701

question is already more rewarding than the study of the problem, and it investigates what it will take to say the project was a success. An effective way to do this is to write a numeric goal statement to show how much change is needed to call it a success. The numeric goal will also be a great way to show progress to both staff and leadership. Example goal statements can be found on The Joint Commission website,[6] which publishes National Patient Safety Goals (NPSGs) each year. The goal should be specific, be measurable, include a deadline, and assign a person or group responsible for meeting the goal.

Once the goal is set, I usually return to all of the people involved. When we go back to the PACU nurses who made all the process changes and report our progress toward the goal, or celebrate improvements, it can be an extremely powerful tool for building a culture of improvement. In contrast, if they make a lot of changes, and no one returns to tell them whether or not it worked, they may stop participating.

SITUATION: Patient survey scores were below threshold, and several patients commented that they lost their belongings after a procedure, which affected their HCAHPS satisfaction scores.

EVIDENCE:

- Raw data from the HCAHPS surveys showed that nearly all patient complaints reported that belongings were lost after a procedure.

- The existing policy was to ask family to hold belongings.

- Interviews with staff revealed that many patients want to keep their cell phone, glasses, and dentures with them, but patient belonging bags are not stocked in the operating wing.

---

6   The Joint Commission (2022). National Patient Safety Goals. Retrieved Aug. 10, 2022, from https://www.jointcommission.org/standards/national-patient-safety-goals/.

- The PACU manager stated that there is no way to order patient belonging bags for PACU to use.

WORKING PROBLEM STATEMENT: PACU staff have no place to put patient belongings.

METHOD OF MEASUREMENT: A review of the data showed that operative patients sampled for HCAHPS surveys represented 5% of the total patient satisfaction scores. Improvement in HCAHPS scores will serve as the method of measurement as it is directly related to the problem.

GOAL STATEMENT: Increase overall patient satisfaction expressed as an overall increase in HCAHPS scores by 5% in the next quarter.

Once a goal statement is written and a method of measurement is determined for the population, the next step is the actual implementation of the solution.

Implementation: Start Making Changes

Once the plan is ready, approval is given, and education is provided, the interventions can be made, and measurement can occur. It is important to keep a detailed log of measurements, as there will be a round of progress reports and presentations to conduct afterwards; the stakeholders involved in the plan all need to know what is happening.

If not done already, the staff who will be directly involved in the actual improvement or change need to hear who is involved, what the project is, what day it will launch, why it is happening, and for how long it will continue as a pilot. I have found from my experience that the "Why?" question is often skipped in the interest of time, but gaining support from staff is usually quite critical to the project. Staff support usually follows a valid explanation, so take time to explain why changes are happening in the most transparent manner possible.

Project Education: Not all projects require in-depth education, but it is a good idea to explore what types of educational
tools (such as webinar platforms or online quiz templates) are
available at your facility. Does the Education Department have
access to a program that would allow you to create a course or
quiz and send it out to specific staff? Does your hospital allow
the use of online form-builders? Does the IT&S Department
have any guidelines about the use of online case studies and
quizzes? Is it possible to offer Continuing Nursing Education
credit for courses, and if so, what course materials are required?
Knowing what resources are available for developing and
measuring education in your facility will make it easier to plan
the use of staff hours in the future.

Part of measurement is setting a deadline for the project: Deadlines
are determined by deciding how long it will take to obtain enough data
to determine if the goal was met. Most measurement deadlines should
occur a few months after the launch date. Of course, every project is
going to have its "honeymoon" period at the outset where the problems
and solutions are fresh in the minds of the staff. But will the solutions
remain effective three months later? Six months later? So it is also
necessary to decide how long the pilot will be studied.

For large projects, it might be wise to launch the project in "waves."
For the launch of Computerized Physician Order Entry (CPOE), we
had several waves based on medical staff designations so that we could
provide personal support to our medical staff: Wave One may have
been the ED physicians, and Wave Two might include hospitalists
and surgeons, for example. Another example is that we wanted to start
the sepsis program ahead of the CMS launch date when they would
announce the specific guidelines, so we started an initial wave (Wave
One) that focused on sepsis recognition training. Once the measure
guidelines were announced by CMS, we could jump right into the
treatment bundle (Wave Two). Dividing a project in this way is based
entirely on the scope of the project.

Regarding personal support, I will say that it helps tremendously to have a number of staff members who are comfortable answering questions about any significant changes and who have direct contact with the QI Department for any issues or problems that arise. These staff members may be called Champions, Super-Users, or anything else that makes sense at your facility, but the role is the same: They are a point of contact for questions and problems. If that type of endorsement is not an option, consider sharing a work phone number for a QI Department staff member or a way to page the Quality Department. This will be used occasionally, and no one needs to be on-call 24/7 to answer questions about a QI project, but the promise of a personal contact will bring palpable relief to the faces of nursing staff, managers, and physicians alike.

Once the launch begins, I go on frequent rounds to the physical site where the change is occurring and talk with staff to check in with them, answer questions, and be available to manage any problems that arise. These rounds also build good will as it shows that QI is owning the project and will help if things go awry. In the example of missing patient items, changes to the policy and paperwork could be made and implemented the same day, and the only pending item would be to measure the effectiveness of that change; there would be no need to divide such a small project into several waves.

Once the project is implemented and live, it is also time to start checking the initial data that comes in those first few days: Keep close tabs on the process and ensure that all gaps are filled, and that data is available. It was not unusual for the Chief Nursing Officer (CNO) to call me out in a morning meeting and ask for a report on one of our pilot projects, so it helps to be prepared to speak about initial data and whether the intended changes are starting to occur.

EXAMPLE IMPLEMENTATION:

SITUATION: Patient survey scores were below threshold and several patients commented that they lost their belongings after a procedure, which affected their HCAHPS satisfaction scores.

EVIDENCE:

- Raw data from the HCAHPS surveys showed that nearly all patient complaints reported that belongings were lost after a procedure.

- The existing policy was to ask family to hold belongings.

- Interviews with staff revealed that many patients want to keep their cell phone, glasses, and dentures with them, but patient belonging bags are not stocked in the operating wing.

- The PACU manager stated that there is no way to order patient belonging bags for PACU to use.

WORKING PROBLEM STATEMENT: PACU staff have no place to put patient belongings.

METHOD OF MEASUREMENT: A review of the data showed that operative patients sampled for HCAHPS surveys represented 5% of the total patient satisfaction scores. Improvement in HCAHPS scores will serve as the method of measurement as it is directly related to the problem.

GOAL STATEMENT: Increase overall patient satisfaction expressed in HCAHPS scores by 5% in the next quarter.

IMPLEMENTATION:

- Update the policy for keeping patient belongings safe during procedures.

- Add patient belonging bags to the supply chain par-stock form.

- Inform staff of the changes to the patient belongings policy in the next staff huddle.

- Collect HCAHPS survey results on an ongoing basis and share findings with leadership and staff.

At this point, the pilot is in full swing, and this is the part where I get nervous: If the wrong problem was selected or some curveball is going to show up, it's going to show up now.

Evaluation: Problem Solved?

The evaluation phase involves more than just monitoring data; it is focused on deciding whether the planned change actually solved the problem statement by a deadline. The evaluation should include data from the initial problem, as well as the pilot proposal and measurement data. All the stakeholders involved in the project will want to hear whether the goal was achieved.

From a data perspective, the evaluation is much like a focused nursing assessment—if you know the patient admitted for respiratory problems, you may not need to do a full gastrointestinal assessment again, but you will certainly be re-evaluating the patient's respiratory status with the start of a new treatment. In the same way, the pilot project is the treatment, and the evaluation phase is the focused nursing assessment. If the goal was not met, ask if the results were unexpected in any way, and whether anything else may have influenced the numbers. Most of the time, if a pilot project is thoughtfully composed, it will have effective results; the ones that need to be revised are usually due to inaccurate problem statements or flawed measurement. When it appears early on that a tool for measurement is not working, the project team will need to decide whether changes should be made during implementation, or for the sake of science should those changes to the pilot be held for more accurate measurement at the end.

The advantage of immediate change is that it is possible to deliver quick, positive changes, and in situations where a pilot project could affect patient safety/harm, that speed in delivery may be important. In contrast, the advantage of patience and accurate measurement is that care is not being delivered based on guesses and estimates during the pilot because each layer of change is carefully measured, and causal relationships can be established. It can be incredibly fruitful to discover how and why a pilot project fails.

I wish that a database of null hypotheses would be created for healthcare research, and it bothers me that only "significant" research gets published; we could learn so much from all the failed experiments, and we would be less likely to repeat failed hypotheses if we took time to study those opposite or inconclusive findings. All that said, I learned a lot from finding what types of audit tools and measurements were ineffective for certain projects. As a rule of thumb, solutions that depend on human beings remembering to do something are more likely to fail (human error), and automated systems and processes are more reliable. Behavioral economist Richard Thaler introduced the idea of the nudge, creating systems that nudge human beings into actions that are beneficial to them, that they would choose to do if asked, but often do not do of their own volition. One example he gives is organ donation, which most people would agree is a good thing to do but were very unlikely to sign up for until states started putting a checkbox on Driver's License renewal forms. This simple nudge increased participation in some states up to 80% of applicants. Nudges tend to be much more effective in increasing buy-in then cudgels like write-ups.[7]

Thus, if the findings show that the pilot was ineffective, rather than jumping to the conclusion that the results are only because of staff failures to follow procedure or complete tasks; ineffectiveness in the process must also be considered and reviewed. The more the reliance on humans remembering to do something can be reduced, the more likely the task is to be completed. The breakdown may have occurred in numerous places, so we will need to investigate contributing factors, look for more research, do more interviews with staff and patients, make a plan for improving the pilot project with ways to further nudge buy-in among staff who are responsible for implementation, and set a fresh launch date and re-evaluation as needed. Project failure should be treated as a significant finding and should be shared with the pilot project committee, but no failure should be presented without understanding why it failed and bringing plans to address the problem the project was created to improve.

At the bedside, this stage would be when the physician gets called

---

7   Thaler, Richard H. (2015). *MisBehaving: The Making of Behavioral Economics.* W. W. Norton & Company: 325-327.

if there are still irregularities in the patient's condition, and additional testing or treatment may be ordered—all based on the nurse's focused assessment. A nurse would not call the physician and waffle on whether the patient's lungs sounded clear or not—the data should be solid before this stage. And the nurse or physician would not immediately blame the patient for being non-compliant with their treatment. But when those additional tests and treatments are carried out, another focused assessment is needed, which may include finding a means to nudge the patient into improved participation in their treatment such as a reminder system for taking medications. And so the cycle continues until the patient improves. In this way, the QI process is just the Nursing Process applied to a project instead of a patient: We would need to revise and repeat the pilot project until the goal is met.

EXAMPLE EVALUATION:

SITUATION: Patient survey scores were below threshold and several patients commented that they lost their belongings after a procedure, which affected their HCAHPS satisfaction scores.

EVIDENCE:

- Raw data from the HCAHPS surveys showed that nearly all patient complaints reported that belongings were lost after a procedure.
- The existing policy was to ask family to hold belongings.
- Interviews with staff revealed that many patients want to keep their cell phone, glasses, and dentures with them, but patient belonging bags are not stocked in the operating wing.
- The PACU manager stated that there is no way to order patient belonging bags for PACU to use.

WORKING PROBLEM STATEMENT: PACU staff have no place to put patient belongings.

METHOD OF MEASUREMENT: A review of the data showed

that operative patients sampled for HCAHPS surveys represented 5% of the total patient satisfaction scores. Improvement in HCAHPS scores will serve as the method of measurement as it is directly related to the problem.

GOAL STATEMENT: Increase overall patient satisfaction expressed in HCAHPS scores by 5% in the next quarter.

IMPLEMENTATION:

- Update the policy for keeping patient belongings safe during procedures,

- Add patient belonging bags to the supply chain par-stock form,

- Inform staff of the changes to the patient belongings policy in the next staff huddle, and

- Collect HCAHPS survey results on an ongoing basis and share findings with leadership and staff.

EVALUATION: HCAHPS patient satisfaction scores improved by 3%, missing the goal of a 5% increase. However, there was an incidental finding that no patient comments mentioned lost belongings, and the Risk Management department states that zero patients filed complaints over missing belongings (compared to several last quarter).

During the evaluation phase, the measurement tool is found to be too broad in scope because so many other factors could influence patient satisfaction. The measurement tool is modified to gather data on the absence of patient complaints about lost belongings. This metric is studied for one year following the project launch.

Since the resolution of the lost belongings problem did not significantly improve the HCAHPS scores, a new project studying factors that could be negatively influencing HCAHPS scores is scheduled to begin.

In true-to-life fashion, our project had some red herrings, some ups and downs, and it ended up spawning a completely new project. But the project is now self-sustaining, and it cost very little to implement. Ironically, the complexity of systemic problems can often result in mixed findings that are actually a clearer picture of our complex reality. The flow of these projects can unveil our inattentional blindness, as well as a host of new opportunities for study. If the QI process sounds intimidating, just remember to keep the problem statement at the front of all decisions; that commitment will make each step clear because doing what is best for the patient is the best thing for the hospital system as well.

PROJECT MANAGEMENT CASE STUDY: SEPSIS BUNDLE COMPLIANCE IN THE ED

After educating staff and launching a new sepsis treatment bundle, we discovered from abstraction data that 30% of our sepsis failures occurred in the ED when the post-treatment evaluation was left incomplete (vital signs were not evaluated after fluid). This step was easy to miss, but it was also a critical step to ensure that the patient was not slipping into shock and that all infection sites were identified and treated. Without the post-treatment evaluation, sepsis mortality could not improve, and our core measure compliance scores were below the minimum threshold. The raw data on our scores showed that this problem was Acute, Big and Costly: A lot of patients' lives were being affected, and it was definitely a top priority for administration because CMS demanded high compliance to receive compensation for care. The next step was to investigate and conduct case studies or "tracers."

Situation: Post-treatment sepsis assessments are often missed in the ED resulting in poor overall bundle compliance scores.

We followed some of our sepsis patients in a tracer and interviewed staff about their experience with the bundle. The ED nurses reported that lack of time and consistency was a major issue—they had to be flexible, and their assignments changed frequently. They said they were trying to follow the sepsis bundle, but after identifying sepsis and starting treatment, it was easy to forget the post-treatment assessment and vital signs at the end of the bundle. Staff confirmed that they were not using the posters on the wall that listed all the required elements of the bundle in fine print, saying "Who has time to read that?"

I had a hunch that there was a system issue here and not an individual-staff performance problem. All of the staff were unable to commit the time to study our Sepsis posters because patient health needs were their immediate concern.

SITUATION: Post-treatment sepsis assessments are often missed in the ED resulting in poor overall bundle compliance scores.

EVIDENCE: There are multiple steps in the sepsis bundle and the final step is the most likely to be missed in the ED. Missed post-treatment assessments represent 30% of SEP-1 compliance failures. Staff report that sepsis bundle posters take too long to review during patient care, and they forget the final steps of the bundle due to rapidly changing assignments.

We knew where to find data on the problem, but would the same data also show improvement? We first needed to identify a problem statement and then select a measurement tool that closely matched the problem.

WORKING PROBLEM STATEMENT: The ED sepsis bundle posters take too long to review, and a more efficient memory tool is needed to improve bundle compliance.

Since bundle compliance was at the center of our problem statement, we decided to use the overall sepsis bundle compliance scores that were already in place from abstraction, and we reviewed the supporting sepsis dashboard to track those scores over time. We determined that the unfamiliar sepsis bundle needed to be related in an obvious and easy way for staff, and our posters were over-complicating it.

So, we needed a way to measure the effects of our actions and goals to show success.

SITUATION: Post-treatment sepsis assessments are often missed in the ED resulting in poor overall bundle compliance scores.

EVIDENCE: There are multiple steps in the sepsis bundle and the final step is the most likely to be missed in the ED. Missed post-treatment assessments represent 30% of SEP-1 compliance failures. Staff report that sepsis bundle posters take too long to review during patient care, and they forget to final steps of the bundle due to frequently changing assignments and lack of familiarity with the sepsis treatment bundle.

WORKING PROBLEM STATEMENT: The ED sepsis bundle posters take too long to review, and a more efficient memory tool is needed to improve bundle compliance.

METHOD OF MEASUREMENT: Data from concurrent and retrospective bundle compliance scores in the ED by month.

GOAL STATEMENT: Improve sepsis bundle compliance by at least 10% by providing an efficient memory tool in the ED to make the treatment bundle more familiar to staff.

We got rid of the small-print posters in the ED, but we debated how to improve those detailed posters with a simpler, faster version. In a casual conversation, one of the QI staff members noted that his kids hardly used words anymore because so many of their conversations occurred via text message using emojis and pictures, which are fast with easy-to-digest images. This realization sparked a new idea that resulted in a new pictograph showing the required steps on a timed arrow: Screening, Labs, Antibiotics, Fluids, Check BP, and a clock set to one-hour. We included a footnote on how to find more detailed information, but this new poster would serve as an at-a-glance reminder for the ED nurses.

Next, it was time to think about what the implementation of our possible solutions would look like. We needed a plan.

SITUATION: Post-treatment sepsis assessments are often missed in the ED resulting in poor overall bundle compliance scores.

EVIDENCE: There are multiple steps in the sepsis bundle and the final step is the most likely to be missed in the ED. Missed post-treatment assessments represent 30% of SEP-1 compliance failures. Staff report that sepsis bundle posters take too long to review during patient care, and they forget to final steps of the bundle due to frequently changing assignments and lack of familiarity with the sepsis treatment bundle.

WORKING PROBLEM STATEMENT: The ED sepsis bundle posters take too long to review, and a more efficient memory tool is needed to improve bundle compliance.

METHOD OF MEASUREMENT: Data from concurrent and retrospective bundle compliance scores in the ED by month.

GOAL STATEMENT: Improve sepsis bundle compliance by at least 10% by providing an efficient memory tool in the ED to make the treatment bundle more familiar to staff.

IMPLEMENTATION:

- Update the sepsis bundle posters in the ED with an efficient pictograph.

- Educate staff on the new posters in the next ED staff huddle.

- Collect concurrent and retrospective abstraction scores on sepsis bundle compliance and share findings with leadership and staff.

RESULTS

Changing the poster helped the ED team improve sepsis bundle compliance by nearly 40% the first week, and it was one of the most rapid turnarounds I have witnessed. Staff were really pleased that we had listened to their needs, and they said the new poster was easy to read at-a-glance in their fast-paced environment. An incidental finding also showed the overall hospital mortality metrics reached zero mortality for severe sepsis patients during the same quarter.

More patients survived sepsis when engagement with the protocol increased in the ED because the poster was easier to read; we solved an "acute," "big," and "costly" problem when we were willing to try something different that was relatively simple and low cost. That's quality for the rest of us.

Chapter 4
Simple Tools

I am addicted to life hacks. I wasn't even looking for a way to plant seedlings in toilet paper rolls, but it worked when I tried it; all my seeds grew. I blame my father. He took carpentry classes a long time ago and now every piece of decent wood gets repurposed into something beautiful and necessary: Old dressers with stuck drawers become custom bookcases, and pantry shelves are refinished to form the base of a storage-ready child's bed. How could I not love the efficiency and beauty of repurposing tools and objects?

Lifehacks for Quality Improvement

Some of the repurposed tools in my arsenal are Quality Improvement (QI) tools that I found to be cumbersome, or else discovered that they just worked better for me when I used them in a different way. Of course, the original tools still have integrity in their own purpose, but there are some tasks in QI that I just had to figure out on my own, and these are the tools I used to do it. This chapter is sort of a "life hacks for QI" collection. If you would like to know about the original evidence-based use of these tools, I would again refer to the sources that do such a good job of explaining them, like the National Association for Healthcare Quality (NAHQ), where a professional and succinct explanation is readily available. But if you're looking for tips and tricks you can use to minimize the effort of accomplishing the giant list of tasks on your QI plate, welcome to my workshop.

Lifehack #1: Hourly Rounding

One useful perspective that may be borrowed from nursing is the practice of purposeful hourly rounding. Research shows that bedside nurses who told patients they would check on them every hour on a handful of critical topics (belongings, pain, etc.) were able to reduce patient anxiety, decrease call-light usage and improve customer satisfaction.[1] Of course, their patients had better outcomes thanks to these nurses' outward-focused mindfulness. This patient tool can also be used to keep a pulse on the facility culture for healthcare improvement. I like to use rounding as a model for staff discussions, asking a couple of open questions, taking notes about any complaints or issues that are brought up, and trying to foster a trusting relationship with staff. Obviously, I would never be able to round on the entire hospital every hour, but the idea of having a routine of connecting frequently with the people affected by our work makes a good deal of sense. I discovered years later that this principle of rounding on the front lines is also called a "Gemba Walk" in Lean Manufacturing methodology.[2] The word "gemba" is derived from the Japanese "gembutsu," which means "the real place." The goal is to not lose sight of the real-life processes we are trying to improve while we examine our data.

If I tried to start working with a problem on paper rather than looking at patient care at the bedside, it could quickly derail the improvement of patient care; I must step back and look at the patient experience over and over again. Focusing on problems instead of patients can be easy to do because there are many organizations marketing their own priorities to the quality team, and many of these priori-

1   Mitchell, M.D.; Lavenberg, J.G.; Trotta, R.; Umscheid, C.A. (2014). Hourly Rounding to Improve Nursing Responsiveness: A Systematic Review. *J Nurs Adm(44)*9, 462-472. DOI: https://doi.org/10.1097/NNA.0000000000000101.

2   *What is a Gemba Walk and why is it important?* (Jan. 17, 2018). Six Sigma Daily. Retrieved Oct. 7th, 2022, from https://www.sixsigmadaily.com/what-is-a-gemba-walk/.

ties require mandatory audits that must be routinely submitted. These audits have a valid reason for existing, but if I lost track of the patient under the paperwork, I would lose my ability to be effective as a health-care improvement professional.

When I round, I know that getting time with staff can be like digging for gold—everyone is busy. I like to watch for the "down times," especially in the Emergency Department, the Operating Room, and the Women's Unit, and try not to distract staff when there are heavy admissions. If I asked them, most staff members would readily tell me when it would be a better time to talk and when they are typically the busiest. Then I came by at least weekly to see how things were going when they had a chance to talk. This practice gives staff a chance to chat about problems, but it also allowed me to keep a pulse on current issues. We don't have call lights for people to report QI problems and solutions; we only have safety and hazard reporting. Why not round before the hazard happens?

The preference is for this rounding habit to be purposeful, but I don't just want to go down my own checklist of priorities. So I am purposefully open-minded on these walks. If someone has a brilliant idea about improving patient care, the only way I am going to hear about it is if I go to the unit and ask them if they have any ideas to improve care. Sometimes they reported problems that we were already working on, and it was rewarding to tell them about the project we were developing and ask if they had any thoughts about it.

An added bonus is that it helps tremendously to have professional contacts in these departments who would guide me away from embarrassing errors if I needed to make changes in their departments at some point. In this respect, "wasting" time in discussions with frontline staff became a tremendous time-saving measure, preventing me from needing to do a complete revision of my project. So try taking a break from the office and check in with the staff providing direct patient care at your facility: You might be surprised by what they say.

Lifehack #2: Motivational Interviewing

I felt nervous when the corporate office of our hospital sent a physician trainer to walk with me (a familiar face) and convince our medical staff to adopt electronic order entry. Federal legislation required physicians to adopt electronic documentation and order sets to improve communication and prevent errors. However, several physicians used typewriters when they went to medical school, and they had no desire to block time for learning a computer application when they could be seeing patients. In addition, some physicians felt embarrassed to be sent "back to school" by this legislation, so it could take a fair bit of persuasion and several visits just to teach the first few steps of logging into the system to a busy and reticent physician.

That morning I had met with the physician trainer for training rounds, and we found one of the surgeons on our list as she was just sitting down to document her patient's post-operative progress. Dr. Brown was nearing retirement and worked part-time, so it was important that we find a way to teach her on the few days she came to the hospital. I greeted Dr. Brown, introduced her to my physician training partner, and explained our purpose.

"I am far too old to be learning these computers, honey," Dr. Brown interrupted my pitch. "I plan to retire soon anyway, so you can just skip me." She waved her hand at me like she was brushing away a fly and chuckled to herself. I continued standing in the cubicle and asked about what she planned to do in retirement. She told me about how she was compiling a book of stories. I said that was wonderful; the nursing staff were all familiar with her storytelling abilities. She collected interesting stories about all aspects of life and shared them whenever she visited patients or dropped by the nurses' station. Her stories delighted us, and she had a knack for gripping our attention.

Next, I asked her how she got it all done: working as a surgeon, devoted mother, and writing a book. She explained her routine and how she identified certain methods that helped her stay sharp and get things done. She told me how much fun it was and how she was learning so much. "As I said, computers are not really my thing, but I knew if I wanted to write this book, I would have to learn how to use a word processor," she explained. "So I read some guides on the internet—yes, I know about the internet," she giggled again. "And I learned how to write on that new-fangled computer."

This was my opening: "I can see that you are a continuous learner. Is that an important characteristic for a physician, too?" I asked.

"Oh yes, we are always learning new techniques for the operating room, or new methods of recovery that will help our patients avoid infection and such. We need to keep studying all the time!" she answered with enthusiasm.

"Well, since you already know how to write on a computer, and you are a continuous learner with effective learning strategies, it will be a cinch for you to learn how to enter these electronic orders. Let me just show you three steps that will be easy for you to learn, and we'll get you checked off on that pending list in the medical staff office."

She laughed and laughed. The physician trainer's eyes widened. We stood there, waiting for her to catch her breath, wondering if she would accept the pitch.

"Oh, you are a clever one!" She finally said, wagging her finger at me. She pushed her glasses up, and said she was ready to try. That day, she learned how to login to the ordering system, how to open a new note, how to place orders from the order sets, and where to find and design custom order sets.

My training partner sat silent the entire time, eyes wide, and arms crossed. When Dr. Brown left with a smile on her face and a promise to let me know when she finished her book, he inquired, "how did you do that? I have never seen someone so reticent to learn become so happy to sit down and train." So what was the marketing trick? Was it just a manipulation? Was it sorcery? Or does it connect to one of the deepest felt needs of contemporary physicians?

I explained that my nursing school allowed our class to participate in a research project using **Motivational Interviewing**. Motivational Interviewing was created by Miller & Rollnick (1991) as a facilitation style that focuses on asking questions.[3] It was developed for counselors to help a person struggling with addictive behavior to identify their own strengths and reasons for change, using the intrinsic beliefs and values that motivate us at an individual level. Basically, it promotes autonomy in decision-making. We all trained and participated in motivational interviewing exercises, and some of my peers even participated in a grant-funded research project using this tool to promote positive health habits.

But the surgeon was not struggling with an addiction, and I was not serving in a counseling role. So what's the connection? I realized during the motivational interviewing training that most of us have a really difficult time listening well. After the training, I made a personal project of developing open-ended questions for first-time conversations, and I practiced asking follow-up questions to help return to subjects I knew my friends and loved ones cared most about. It started as a way to show that I cared about my family and friends, but I soon realized that if I could ask good questions and let someone really talk, I could learn a lot from others.

The thing that I love about motivational interviewing is that it highlights the fact that everyone has overcome some problem at some point in time: Everyone has some level of resilience. Even babies struggle to walk and talk but they don't give up trying. We are naturally motivated to overcome difficulties, and anytime we are willing to try, there is potential for growth. People are often ambivalent about learning or trying to meet a goal because they do not think they will be successful (or that it will really help), but by asking questions about previous successes and how they overcame past difficulties, those same coping skills can beat a new problem as soon as we discover the motivation to change. It is deeply empowering.

I knew that Dr. Brown was a continuous learner filled with curios-

---

3   Miller, W.R.; Rollnick, S. (1991). Motivational Interviewing: Preparing people to change addictive behavior. *J of Community & Applied Soc Psych. 2(4).* 299-300. https://doi.org/10.1002/casp.2450020410.

ity, skill, and optimism, so it was not hard to ask growth questions. By simply asking her to tell me about herself and following up on the barrier she identified, we both found the tools needed to learn the new task. It's about respecting someone else's decisions and autonomy and asking questions to help them remember all the times in the past that they have solved problems. At that point, they can make a choice to try or not try, but the barriers are gone, and the plan is tailored to the individual.

For example, if you had to think back to some of the most difficult trials in your life, what characteristics helped you solve the problem and persevere? Who were the people that supported you or believed in you? Where did you go for help when you got stuck? The answers to those questions might be the solution to a current problem if you can find a way to rally the same characteristic, support system, or resource. In Dr. Brown's case, the barrier to learning was not so much a disagreement with computerized order entry—she had no problem with computers and believed it would improve patient safety to eliminate handwriting. The true barrier was that she felt it was nearly impossible for her to learn new technology at this stage of her life and career. It was as if she believed that the medical world was moving on without her, and she was powerless to stop it.

Powerlessness is exactly how people would describe their feelings when struggling with addiction. In medicine, we usually talk about patients who are powerless, which is why we have things like informed consent—to empower patients in their medical decisions. When a patient feels empowered, they have better clinical outcomes.[4] Motivational Interviewing empowers patients by listening and asking questions about personal successes and it facilitates a way for people—even physicians—to solve their own problems using the coping skills that worked in the past. I believe this is more respectful than telling someone

4   Werbrouk, A.; Swinnen, E.; et al (2018). How to empower patients? A systematic review and meta-analysis. *Translational Behavioral Medicine*. 8(5). 660-674. https:// academic.oup.com/tbm/article-abstract/8/5/660/5048802.

how they should solve a problem, or refusing to listen because they have no choice, and that is why I use motivational interviewing in my work. We have mandatory regulations, but we have room to find new ways of implementing them. So why not discuss the plan with the people implementing it? What barriers do they see and how have they overcome them in the past?

I should mention that this facilitation tool doesn't always work quickly. Sometimes, the physician just flatly disagrees with the change itself. Sometimes it takes a lot more discussion to alleviate concerns about the latest research and regulatory standards. Other times, it's just a really bad time in the physician's life and they are simply not ready for something new—all of their coping resources are already in use, and there is no room for another challenge. But I've learned that listening is valuable regardless, and asking good questions that help others discover things about themselves can be an invaluable skill. The goal is to build relationships and cultivate understanding, not to manipulate people or force them into doing something. And since I try to cultivate this quality in myself, I have to respect the physicians that question me about new standards—it shows that they care and that is a good thing.

I fully realize that it is unconventional to apply a counseling method to the staff-physician relationship, but it makes sense: I have heard so many physicians express frustration that everyone tells them how to practice medicine (government, hospital oversight, researchers, insurance providers, etc.). When they were studying leadership during all those years of education, they were taught that they would be granted a degree of independence and autonomy: that they would use their best judgment to make decisions even when all of the information was not necessarily available. But instead, they are on the phone arguing about whether their treatment decision is "medically necessary" with someone who typically has less education and clinical training. No wonder they feel disrespected. That is why I believe that listening and facilitation is so important. If I want to have a respectful conversation with the medical staff and provide the independence they need to do their best work, I need to listen respectfully, and that doesn't always come naturally when my career will rise or fall based on compliance scores. Many physicians do not believe anyone is listening to them, and they are often exhausted from the demands of their schedule. But thoughtfully listening and being respectful will improve the hospital culture itself.

For more information about Motivational Interviewing, see Miller and Rollnick's initial article on the technique, "Motivational Interviewing: Preparing people to change addictive behavior" published in 1991, or feel free to search the plethora of journal archives on the topic since then for a more recent example.

Lifehack #3: Mortality Review

I once attended a webinar by a major research hospital on the topic of Mortality Review. When they shared how they had requested several autopsies for the sake of science, I suddenly felt like the lost orphan of QI. If I mentioned such an extravagant request to my own leadership team, they would have a good laugh about it. I wondered if that was really required to understand mortality review? While I learned the general principles and benefits of mortality review from that webinar, I was intimidated because I knew that a request for an elective autopsy at a community hospital would raise some eyebrows. We did not have a research budget or team of scientists to analyze the data. I would say that most hospitals do not conduct an in-depth mortality review precisely for this reason—it seems like an extravagant, "big research hospital" method that does not really affect the real-world problems of the local facility. Some facilities with specialized programs will focus on a specific diagnosis, like heart disease or pneumonia, and pull those patients to see if they received all the recommended treatments or care bundles, but it is still common to delay or cut even these focused mortality reviews when time and staff are limited.

Hospitals do submit mandatory electronic data on mortality for specific diagnoses, but it is all automated with the CMS electronic portal, and it is frequently untouched and unreviewed at the local level. Initially, these required diagnoses are often selected by CMS as a 30-day mortality review, for example, or by a quality survey tool like Leapfrog™, and they are primarily based on discharge diagnosis coding.

I would like to clearly state that mortality review does not need to be an extravagant project; mortality reviews are one of the single best ways to identify significant problems at a facility without expensive research or fancy databases. If there are budget cuts to the data analytics fund, focusing on mortality review may be the single most affordable and effective solution you can find.

Why is that?

When I struggle with setting priorities, my patient-focused tools always bring me back to mortality review because it focuses on the ultimate patient outcome: Survival. When patients come to the hospital, they typically plan on leaving alive, and that is why mortality review is a fast way to sort a large number of patient charts down to the ones that need QI attention. We know that every patient who died was either expected to die, or not. Quality healthcare should always be about the patient, and mortality review is an effective way to see if the patient achieved what they wanted in coming to the hospital.

So what is involved in doing mortality review, and do I really need to budget for elective autopsies? At the most basic level, mortality review starts with sorting the charts of patients who died at the facility over a specific timeframe and determining whether the death was "expected" or "not expected." This stage is also called a "preliminary review." The charts can be easily sorted out by discharge code and date, so retrieval of the data is simple. There is no blame assigned, and there is no requirement to follow-up because it is not a litigation exercise where care needs to be defended—it is an exploration for the sake of learning.

When I conduct a mortality review, I use this list and mark the charts "E" or "NE" for expected/not expected deaths. Once that list is created, I add a column to make additional notes in a more systematic review. For the not expected (NE) deaths, I write down anything I found interesting, any potential errors, whether the appropriate protocols were followed, and any hospital-acquired conditions. I continue to avoid assigning any type of blame to any person, group, or unit during this preliminary review—I don't want to jump to conclusions before I have fully reviewed the case. However, after a thorough review is complete, I would notify the Risk Management Department of any potential negligence or medical errors if they were noted. Once I gathered data about patients by diagnosis, the next step was to exclude "expected" deaths and create notes about each of the "not expected" deaths. Are there any repeated problems? Does any trend stand out? What do they have in common and what is different? I then use these observations to put together a case study with evaluations about care and any recommendations revealed from the data.

That's it.

There are certainly more involved and more paper-heavy versions of mortality review for those individuals with the time and budget to do so. But as I mentioned at the beginning of this chapter, these are my "life hacks" versions of QI tools, and this is the mortality review that helped me focus my programs and make important decisions about patient care priorities. For hospitals facing a discouraging amount of work in reactive audits, for example, I would recommend stepping back from the numbers and meetings to think about what would make the biggest difference for patients right now: What would help more patients survive? If the answer is not apparent, start with mortality reviews to find what will make a difference for real people, and the numbers will follow.

Because of the information gleaned in mortality review, we were able to launch inter-departmental projects that increased the hospital's performance and revenue. Prior to the mortality review, we had no idea the problem existed. It is also a lot like the mystery books and detective shows that I love—Mortality review is all about solving mysteries. Opportunities for improvement are surprisingly apparent in a review of deceased patient charts, and it is one of the simplest, most affordable, low-tech ways to see problems and trends.

It is so important for me to leave work at the end of the day knowing that I made a meaningful and positive difference. Finding at least one small thing that I could improve helped me wade through the pile of audits on my desk, and I usually found those golden nuggets in mortality review. Eventually, those proactive, small improvements decreased my audits and helped me reach other goals on my wish-list for improvement.

Lifehack #4: Root Cause Analysis

By far one of my favorite tools in the QI life hacks toolkit is the Root Cause Analysis (RCA). The RCA is a way to find the source of a problem and it is typically used to dig deeper on incidents of patient harm or errors that occur in the patient safety sector. It can also be used for improvement, and it is most effective when the people who are part of the process are part of the RCA. So, if you need to solve a problem with patient belongings missing in PACU, be sure to include a clinician from the PACU in the RCA meeting.

The first step in the RCA is a step that I never thought about before studying QI methods: Describe what is normal. Only the people who do these tasks every day know what normal looks like, yet we often fail to ask about the normal workflow when we are digging into an abnormal incident. What processes are already in place and what would the normal steps look like? Ask detailed questions about where things are stored, why someone is called for a certain duty, what is the availability of phones on that unit to page the physician, whether a document needs to be printed or whether it is available as a pre-printed packet—all the details. Ask what is the normal workflow, and why is that the normal process? This line of questioning leads to an analysis of all the potential contributing factors. Does the printer often jam? Is it difficult to reach key players in the process? Where are the tools located for checking the temperature of that refrigerator? What are all the common problems that tend to go wrong in this process? There will be a wide array of contributing factors that may be human factors, environmental, or process related. Write them all down in a second column (after the normal process column) and do not organize them, yet.

Once the "normal" workflow is described and a list of contributing factors is available, the next step is to describe the problem. What could or did go wrong in this specific incident? Keep it simple and allow the problem statement to flow from the contributing factors list. There can be more than one problem statement, and it should be process-focused rather than people-focused because the purpose is not to assign blame but to discover opportunities in a flawed process.

Once a problem statement is available, the final step is to identify potential solutions. I continue to be shocked by how clear those solutions can become once all of the details are written down about the existing process next to the problem at hand. The potential cause of a problem becomes apparent, and the solution is somewhere in the opposite direction. Try to find solutions that do not depend on human behavior, but look for ways to improve the situation, environment, timing, and availability of resources so that the ideal process can be repeated without human memory or effort (because people have enough to think about).

By the end of the RCA, there will be actionable solutions that can be discussed with the team. An action plan can be created based on the QI Process (see previous chapter) and change can be measured and re-evaluated for lasting improvement. (*See Table 4.1*)

One of my unconventional applications of a Root Cause Analysis is with abstraction accuracy results. If I discovered any Inter-Rater Reliability (IRR) or Validation results with a mismatch, I would whip out my RCA tool and investigate the normal abstraction process, contributing factors, identify problems, and make an improvement action plan. This was a great alternative to personalized write-ups, and it was a great way to demonstrate thorough analysis of the problem.

One example from these projects was when we discovered the radiology contractor who read and reported our imaging results worked in a different time zone, and that difference could affect stroke

TABLE 4.1 - EXAMPLE ROOT CAUSE ANALYSIS: MISSING PATIENT BELONGINGS

NORMAL	CONTRIBUTING FACTORS	PROBLEMS	SOLUTIONS
Patient belongings placed on the bed prior to procedure	Patients do not give belongings to family or put in safe because they want cell phone after surgery to place calls	Need to choose and communicate about the best place for belongings	Recommend safe or family members as the best place for belongings
Belongings stay with sedated patient	Patient is positioned for procedure and belongings must move off the bed	Need a safe place to put belongings without disrupting procedure.	Bed has a hook for patient belonging bags and incomplete IV medications
PACU staff leave belongings on the bed until patient awakes. Hand-off does not include belongings. Difficult to reach pre-op and intra-op staff to ask about belongings.	No belonging bags available pre-op or intra-op, lost time searching for missing items in PACU, unable to confirm from report on whether belongings are missing or whether patient is confused from anesthesia	Belonging bags not included in floor stock list for pre-op requisitions and belongings not typically mentioned at hand-off	Request belonging bags be added to floor stock in pre-op and include belongings in hand-off template

abstraction. When we explored the normal process of abstraction and reviewed the differences with the team, we found that the note was reported in the contractor's time rather than the facility's time zone (which should be abstracted). After the RCA, we carried out an action plan that included an educational review of the error and a solution tool for abstraction staff to convert time zones. This was a non-disciplinary finding because the error was not due to abstractor negligence, but rather a lack of knowledge in the reporting process for electronic radiology notes. It was a helpful discovery, and the abstraction team was key to the development of the action plan.

So whenever the source of a problem is unclear (even if it is not necessarily a clinical problem), I like using the Root Cause Analysis to gain a thorough understanding of the problem and include other staff members in the improvement process.

Lifehack #5: Barrier Analysis

There are so many quality tools and templates that are wonderful, but when I discovered the Barrier Analysis, it was love at first sight. I immediately pulled out a notebook and started applying it to several of the problems in my head. The original Barrier Analysis is part of a behavioral change methodology used in public health. It was originally created by Tom Davis to study barriers to water sanitation among Haitian workers in the Dominican Republic. The Dominican Republic shares an island with Haiti, and for the most part Haitians are a marginalized group in the Dominican Republic.[5] Davis noted that Haitian sugar cane cutters (known locally as *braceros*) were not utilizing best practices when it came to water sanitation even after his team had taught them how to clean their water for drinking, and when he

---

5   *A Stolen Trombone, Barrier Analysis and Isaiah 65 – A chat with Tom Davis – World Vision's New Global Lead for Sustainable Health* (Feb. 9, 2018). World Vision International. Retrieved Sept. 8, 2022, from https://www.wvi.org/article/stolen-trombone-barrier-analysis-and-isaiah-65-chat-tom-davis-world-visions-new-global-lead.

asked their Dominican supervisors why the *braceros* were not cleaning their water, he got answers like "they're lazy, they can't understand the message," and other answers that referred to presumed human flaws.

Davis knew there had to be more to the story, so he developed a survey to analyze the situation that eventually became known as the Barrier Analysis. It turned out that the *braceros* wanted to clean their water and knew how, but they could not afford the bleach at the company store. *Braceros* were brought into the Dominican Republic to cut sugar cane, but their importation left them indebted to the companies that employed them, and the interest on that debt was structured in a way that it could never be repaid, much like American coal miners in historical Appalachia. Every bit of income they had went back to the company for food and shelter, and there was not enough left over for bleach or gallon-sized containers for cleaning water. The barrier did turn out to be a cultural one, just a culture of racism and human abuse, which took years to rectify.

While there will hopefully never be a human-rights atrocity at the root of issues affecting your facility, the Barrier Analysis is a very useful tool for uncovering unseen causes of those issues. If, for example, the goal was to increase hand-washing compliance in a hospital, the barrier analysis might be used to figure out why some people do not wash their hands consistently—maybe the sinks are too far away, or the soap runs out and cannot be refilled easily? Overall, inconvenience might be the chief reason why handwashing is lower than desired and a new marketing program for handwashing with the message "it's easy to get sick" might focus on the inconvenience of illness, coupled with better access to soap refills to improve the compliance numbers quite a bit. Maybe staff feel overwhelmed and overworked, and hand washing seems like a lower priority than getting those eight patient baths completed in the next two hours. This issue will almost certainly not be the stereotypical reasons that spring to mind without investigating and analyzing data about the situation. While I've never worked in water sanitation in the Caribbean or designed a handwashing program for a hospital, I think the barrier analysis is useful because we are all really good at offering excuses for why we cannot or will not change.

And speaking of a break from reality, in my utopian view of my working self, I always complete all of my work projects in a timely manner. But in reality, I keep coming up with excuses for why I can't have my utopia. So then how do I know which excuses are legitimate and which ones are just me being unreasonable? That's where a personal Barrier Analysis can be helpful. So while the true barrier analysis tool is more in-depth and focused on public health, I like using a super-simple version for time management because I can exercise all my skills at making great excuses. One of those excuses was that I could not find the priority task in my schedule (and I certainly should not start without finding the priority, right?).

Time management is a huge deal in healthcare, and sometimes when the projects stack up, the workload can feel overwhelming. Everything on the list affects patient care, and anything I missed could potentially result in lower quality care for a real person in my community. That can be a lot of pressure. So, rather than feel anxious about the volume of work, I used the Barrier Analysis tool to prioritize my schedule.

So how does the Barrier Analysis work?

In a spreadsheet column, I write down all of the tasks I need to complete and clear my head of all the things I worry I might forget. This step can take quite a while, and it should be thorough. I put down "check email daily" on the same list as "achieve zero mortality for severe sepsis" and "educate community about antibiotic stewardship." You can imagine this list gets pretty lengthy with both mundane tasks and hard-to-reach stretch goals. Incidentally, my barrier analysis list has always been a good thing to have on hand when my supervisor starts asking whether I have room on my plate for a few side projects. This long list of duties and goals helps track my work and communicates details about my value to the company.

Once the list of goals is complete, I would add a new column to list every barrier that prevented me from meeting each goal, one-by-one. This stage requires some time to really think about what it would take to complete the project. Does it take time, or does it cost money? Is it difficult to rally support among key players? I wrote down everything that prevented success in achieving the stated goals. The next step is to prioritize each barrier by how important the goal is, and how difficult it would be to accomplish. At this point, I often chose to score the priority level and color-code the difficulty of my barriers: green is simple, yellow is moderate, red is difficult, purple requires a miracle, etc. Feel free to customize your own analysis according to preference. It should be a simple list with a score for difficulty, a score for importance, and room to assign a priority number when finished.

The final step is to find the highest priority tasks with a specific deadline. I like to identify the tasks that are easy and important (also known as "low-hanging fruit") because they can be done quickly and provide a good return. For example, I found that sitting down and editing a pending order set would likely improve our compliance scores significantly, but it would only take a day or two to complete my portion of the task. Once the priorities are selected, I can develop an action plan for the top priority and start chiseling away at those goals.

In practice, I usually breakdown the difficult and important tasks into smaller steps to make them more achievable. That way, I can make steady progress toward the final goal. An example for this type of goal was the community education project. I took the goal of educating the community about antibiotic stewardship, and broke it down into:

1. develop community education in laymen's terms for non-clinical students

2. identify opportunities to teach with the public relations and marketing department

3. set a specific and achievable goal for the number of teaching sites to visit

4. measure comprehension at each site with a post-class survey

I mentioned above that a deadline needs to be established, and I would like to explain that setting time-dependent goals is not an arbitrary activity. As much as my idealistic self would like to believe that I will accomplish all of those great goals without a deadline, I know that it is a false assumption. If I go to the trouble of making a color-coded, scored list of my pending duties, there had better be a due date for those tasks or else I will just have a pretty, but useless list.

The Barrier Analysis tool can be used for a variety of problems. I have also used this process to analyze IT Access requests. When combined with a Gantt Flowchart to watch for bottlenecks in the process, it worked marvelously well. Quality tools are used in many different fields, from auto manufacturing to software development, and I thoroughly enjoy applying those tools in unusual ways. The chance to be both creative and analytical is a wonderful benefit to healthcare QI as a professional field. (*See Table 4.2*)

Lifehack #6: Length of Stay Index (LOSI)

In nursing school, one of my instructors taught us the principle of Discharge Barrier Rounds, where the charge nurse, primary nurse, and case manager rounded on the unit to discuss what was keeping each patient from safely discharging home. We talked about any case management barriers such as durable medical equipment needs and transportation, or whether their antibiotics could be completed under home health care, and whether nursing had reported the patient's constipation to the surgeon so that orders could be written to prevent an ileus. I quickly realized that this concept was completely in-line with what most patients really want. It is the number one question every clinician hears a thousand times a day: "When can I go home?"

Since my nursing school days, I have learned more about this process. Now I understand that Case Managers and Clinical Documentation Integrity (CDI) specialists review a variety of metrics based on CMS data on the expected length of stay by diagnosis code. One of my favorites among those metrics is the Length of Stay Index (LOSI), which is similar to the mortality index in that it compares actual length of stay (LOS) measured in days and compared to the national average LOS for that diagnosis. A LOSI score less than 1 indicates a shorter than average length of stay, and a score greater than 1 means the patient is staying in the hospital longer than expected. The national average LOS is listed with the Diagnosis Related Group (DRG) codes published by CMS, and the hospital typically uses this data for case management and CDI workflows—because an increased length of stay can be an indicator of things like increased cost, barriers found in the social determinants of health assessment, a difficult discharge placement, or a mismatch between the documented diagnosis and the patient's condition (the patient is in septic shock but the diagnosis is for cholecystitis without complications, for example). An extended LOS is associated with increased cost, and it is better to know about these barriers early in the encounter rather than later.

Some hospitals pull this data into their Electronic Medical Record (EMR) where physicians and nurses can anticipate discharge needs and collaborate with the interdisciplinary team. However, many hospitals do not routinely communicate this information to clinical staff. A review of the LOSI score for each patient could help hospitals prepare discharge paperwork in advance (obtaining appointments prior to the weekend, for example), as well as identify patients with additional needs when the LOSI is higher than expected.

I would love to see this metric integrated in the electronic patient list itself, where the EMR could pull the LOSI automatically and display it for the entire team: Patient names could turn green when they are within 48 hours of expected discharge, or their name could turn yellow when they are overdue for discharge, for example. Those patients who are over the expected timeframe could be reviewed by the care team to solve barriers and help the patient get the care that they need in a timely manner.

Regardless of my EMR dreams, excess LOS is going to continue to be on the administrative radar because it inadvertently impacts staffing—when nurses are caring for a patient who could have gone home

TABLE 4.2 – EXAMPLE BARRIER ANALYSIS: SEPSIS COORDINATOR TIME MANAGEMENT					
GOAL	**BARRIERS**	**DIFFICULTY**	**IMPORTANCE**	**PRIORITY**	**DEADLINE**
Clean email inbox	Time it takes to read long newsletters	Easy	Moderate	3	Weekly
Teach community about sepsis	Time to create new curriculum; finding opportunities	Moderate	Low	4	End of month
Edit sepsis order set	Time to review and edit order set	Easy	High	1	End of week
Zero severe sepsis mortality score	Support from medical staff for delivery of fluids	Difficult	High	2	End of quarter

the day before, that nurse is unable to take a new admission. I recommend integrating the LOSI into the daily administrative review to ensure that patients receive timely care, and clinicians receive support for solving unique problems. I believe this is an action item that would be appropriate for the Quality Department to champion since a successful discharge affects multiple quality indicators as well.

Lifehacks - Summary

The world of QI is replete with some amazing tools that were created by inquiring minds who were just trying to make their work turn out better. Whether it is a carpenter repurposing a broken dresser into a custom bookcase or adopting the Barrier Analysis to sort through my projects at work, there is a simple beauty in finding a tool that fits the problem. Beyond the tools and ideas in this chapter, QI allows me to practice continuous improvement on a personal level: I continue to study and learn new things that I can apply in my professional work every day, and I find that I sincerely enjoy hearing from other professionals about their clever ideas and simple solutions. Perhaps these tools are helpful to you; perhaps you have an idea that will help me improve patient care. That's part of the reason I created the PorterQI community at https://PorterQI.com. We can help so many people when we spend time learning from each other and continue sharing ideas for improvement.

But while PorterQI is a great resource for professionals to help each other, far be it from me to reinvent the wheel when there are so many existing organizations out there that are working toward Quality Improvement in the healthcare industry. Let's take a look at some of the most notable quality organzations in the industry.

Organizations That Help With Quality Improvement

When I was a brand-new quality analyst just starting out in abstraction, I had no idea there were organizations with resources to help me in my work. I also met a significant number of QI professionals who were embarrassed to admit that they did not know where to find the official guidelines, the original specifications manual, or even the organization that wrote the rules—they were trained on the job to just click on the vendor tool link and were unaware of any other resources.

Later in my career, I discovered a myriad of resources with templates, tools, and expert courses applying QI principles to real-world practice. I also found the original guidelines on federally recognized regulatory websites. These organizations and resources are for everyone. They are not just for elite research scientists, or for professionals with decades of experience. They are meant for you and me at whatever level of experience we have when we come to the table.

I wished that someone had told me that these resources were available; I literally designed every poster, cut and laminated badge-sized cheat-sheets, drafted presentations, and manually typed spreadsheets, only to find out that much of the material was readily available online for free download. If this is your experience as well (usually because the budget required it), just try to contain your excitement as we tour a literal outpouring of free downloads, coursework, professional contacts, and other incredibly helpful tools available from these organizations. The regulatory organizations are discussed in more detail in the **Abstraction & Public Reporting** chapter, but the list below covers a selection of the organizations that are dedicated to help QI professionals improve healthcare. Please note that this list is not even remotely exhaustive—there are so many other organizations and resources that I could not begin to fit them all in a single list, but these are some of my favorites, and they are not in any kind of priority order:

The Institute for Healthcare Improvement (IHI)

ABOUT: Founded about thirty years ago, the IHI uses improvement science to improve patient outcomes globally. They create innovative solutions that are shared in educational courses, an annual conference, and "White Papers" that share findings and ideas online.[6] The IHI also provides certification in patient safety.

PROS: The IHI offers first-class education in healthcare improvement, including base courses that provide sample tools and worksheets to apply quality concepts to real facilities and projects. There are advanced topics as well as basic courses available in QI with practical tools. The educational quality of the coursework is first-class with simulations, videos, case studies, and professionally-designed worksheets to support the course content. Recent materials also focus on equity in healthcare, which could be helpful to a diversity and equity professional.

CONS: The IHI membership fee is prohibitively expensive, and material useful to improving patient outcomes with science-backed clinical guidance, worksheets, and templates are almost ten years old. Material developed more recently prioritizes environmental, social, and governance changes (such as roles and committees) rather than patient outcomes. Of course, as CMS develops new guidelines on health equity and enacts mandatory reporting of demographics, IHI's work in this area may be an important data lake for the healthcare quality professional or facility manager looking to improve ESG scores, depending on how those measures will be required to be reported. [7]

---

6   The Institute for Healthcare Improvement (2022). About. Retrieved July 31, 2022, from http://www.ihi.org/about/Pages/default.aspx.

7   The Centers for Medicare and Medicaid Services (2022). CMS Framework for Health Equity 2022-2032. Retrieved July 31, 2022, from https://www.cms.gov/files/document/cms-framework-health-equity-2022.pdf.

The Agency for Healthcare Research and Quality (AHRQ)

ABOUT: The AHRQ is a federal agency charged with improving patient safety and quality in the United States healthcare system. They use research to develop tools and data for improvement to help patients, professionals, and policymakers make decisions.[8] AHRQ also publishes Quality Indicators (QIs) and Patient Safety Indicators (PSIs) for hospitals to highlight potential quality improvement areas.[9]

PROS: The AHRQ focuses on practical problems such as healthcare-acquired infections, communication barriers, discharge delays, pressure ulcers, and other topics that are directly relevant to patient care in healthcare facilities. There is also an extensive database of national healthcare statistical reports available free of charge. AHRQ is an essential stop for any research project.

CONS: The breadth of research and data available through AHRQ is difficult to work through. A list of "trending topics" on the website includes multiple, massive, game-changing projects that are all applicable to healthcare facilities, so it can be overwhelming to decide where to start—but the Clinical Quality Indicators page would be a good first step.

---

8 Agency for Healthcare Research and Quality (n.d.). About. Retrieved March 9, 2022, from https://www.ahrq.gov/cpi/index.html.

9 Agency for Healthcare Research and Quality (n.d.). Quality Indicators. Retrieved March 9, 2022, from https://qualityindicators.ahrq.gov/Default.aspx.

The National Association for Healthcare Quality (NAHQ)

ABOUT: NAHQ (pronounced Nay-Q) focuses on advancing the profession of healthcare quality. They aim to prepare the workforce to lead and advance quality in healthcare. This organization publishes the respected Journal for Healthcare Quality, hosts a national conference, and offers an accredited certification in healthcare quality called the Certified Professional in Healthcare Quality (CPHQ) credential. Recently, they also developed a competency framework for the QI professional role, and there is an online assessment for identifying opportunities for professional development.[10] I took the survey and was pleased to see a scored results page listing my strengths and weaknesses with content suggestions for further study. This assessment could be used to guide corporate training as well as personal development goals.

PROS: The website is simple and easy to read, and the fees are affordable. The CPHQ exam is a golden ticket to fluently navigating the QI profession, and the eligibility requirements are minimal. When I consider the knowledge gaps I had when I started in QI (and the needs expressed by other professionals), I believe NAHQ is on the cutting edge because they are delivering practical, high-quality materials that are immediately relevant to my work.

CONS: The simple, easy-to-navigate website comes at a cost as detailed descriptions are sparse and do not reference a way to uncover additional details on subjects. The Journal of Healthcare Quality and CPHQ network are only available with a membership at an additional fee.

The National Academy of Medicine (NAM)

ABOUT: Originally chartered as the National Academy of Sciences in 1863, the NAM is a non-profit, non-governmental organization

---

10   National Association for Healthcare Quality (2022). About. Retrieved Aug. 22, 2022, from https://nahq.org/about-nahq/.

devoted to advancing science to improve health. Formerly known as the Institute of Medicine (IOM), NAM published a report in 2000, *To Err Is Human: Building a Safer Health System*,[11] which documented serious patient safety problems in the United States healthcare system. Specifically, this document reported that while public trust in the healthcare system was high, medical errors were one of the top causes of death in the nation, which is still the case today. The importance of this report is what puts the NAM on my favorites list.

PROS: The whistle-blowing document, *To Err Is Human*, is pivotal to the field of quality improvement and should be read by every QI professional.

CONS: The NAM is an elite network that has recently been distracted from the ongoing issue of medical errors to pursue topics in climate change and health culture. Since there are many organizations focused on climate change, and too few focused on reducing medical errors, I am concerned that this leading cause of mortality will continue to abound in the industry without solutions.[12]

The National Quality Forum (NQF)

ABOUT: NQF is "A non-profit, nonpartisan, membership-based organization that works to catalyze improvements in healthcare."[13] This organization is focused on measurement science to provide standardized tools capable of adjusting to change in the health system. NQF designs and reviews healthcare measures for CMS and sets standards for national quality initiatives. This is the organization that decides whether we will have heart disease measures or sepsis bundles as our

---

11   Kohn, L.T.; Corrigan, J.M.; Donaldson, M.S. (Eds.) (2000). *To Err is Human: Building a Safer Health System*. National Academies Press.

12   National Academy of Medicine (n.d.). The Climate Grand Challenge. Retrieved Aug. 22, 2022, from https://nam.edu/programs/climate-change-and-human-health/.

13   National Quality Forum (2022). About. Retrieved March 8, 2022, from https://www.qualityforum.org/About_NQF/.

next measure of QI performance.

PROS: The topics discussed are practical, including things like mortality review and Health Information Technology. NQF presents science-driven standards with well-documented evidence, and serves as an incubator for quality measure development. Following NQF projects would be a good way to remain current in research and data analysis. The website shows what quality measures are being considered for the future, and individuals can even comment on them during the public comment period.

CONS: It could be difficult for an individual to join and organizational NQF membership fees are based on a scale. The organizations future-oriented mission does not have an immediate effect on issues facing quality professionals in the moment.

American Society for Quality (ASQ)

ABOUT: Based in Milwaukee, Wisconsin, ASQ provides professional training, certifications, and publications in the field of QI.[14] Compared to other organizations, the variety of topics offered at conferences and events are more diverse and innovative, including topics in technology innovation with artificial intelligence, women in leadership, and management of change and disruption in the 21st century.

PROS: ASQ is an excellent source for resources and the membership is reasonably priced. A wide array of Six Sigma courses are available, as well as courses and reading lists geared toward new quality professionals.

CONS: Individual courses and certifications are billed as a separate fee, and while membership offers a discount, they are still expensive enough that individuals are somewhat out-priced by corporate and group training.

---

14   American Society for Quality (2022) About. Retrieved March 8, 2022, from https://asq.org/about-asq.

American Hospital Association (AHA)

ABOUT: The American Hospital Association was founded in 1898 to represent hospitals and healthcare networks for the purpose of advocacy in national health policy formation, as well as providing a source of information on health care issues and trends, such as workforce management and cybersecurity.[15] AHA lobbyists represent the needs of members in national health policy discussions at the executive, legislative, regulatory, and judicial arenas.

PROS: This is a great source for current news about the healthcare industry. Innovative hospitals are featured in articles, and lobbyist statements to Congress are posted for public viewing. There is generally more information about the cost and details of innovative ventures, as well as any changes in the business side of healthcare. Membership is not required to view articles, and the information that is shared for free in the AHA News site would typically carry a steep fee at most other healthcare executive news sources.

CONS: The intended audience is the healthcare executive with a bias toward cost management and logistics.

American Society for Healthcare Risk Management (ASHRM)

ABOUT: The American Society for Healthcare Risk Management is focused on providing the safest, low-risk care for patients, without excessive cost. It is a professional membership affiliate of the American Hospital Association for safe and trusted care, and includes other professional fields such as legal professionals, insurance providers, and hospital finance.[16] They offer the Certified Professional in Healthcare

---

15 The American Hospital Association (2022). About the AHA. Retrieved Oct. 24, 2022 from https://www.aha.org/about.

16 American Society for Health Care Risk Management (2022). About. Retrieved Aug. 2, 2022, from https://www.ashrm.org/about-1.

Risk Management (CPHRM) credential as well as webinars with continuing education credits in patient safety and risk management.

PROS: They provide an authoritative guide to current issues in patient safety with a helpful legal and financial component to the education. There are "foundations" courses for new professionals, which is always appreciated.

CONS: The cross-disciplinary risk management focus occasionally obscures the clinical quality perspective, but it is still a useful supplement to gain perspective on critical patient safety topics.

The Sepsis Alliance

ABOUT: The Sepsis Alliance is a non-profit charity dedicated to battling sepsis.[17] It is the leading sepsis organization in the United States and was founded in 2007 to raise awareness about sepsis in the general public as well as in healthcare facilities.

PROS: As a new sepsis coordinator, I joined a forum through the Sepsis Alliance that was for professionals involved in building and maintaining sepsis programs. I cannot express how helpful it was to be able to discuss problems in a live, professional environment. There is also a variety of patient and staff education materials on their website with helpful graphics and videos, and they do an excellent job of maintaining current scientific evidence on the subject while not neglecting the human side. They offer materials for focused populations such as pediatrics.

CONS: While the message is similar, the Sepsis Alliance is not connected with CMS and cannot serve as a substitute for SEP-1 core measure guidelines.

---

17   The Sepsis Alliance (2022). About. Retrieved July 23, 2022, from https://www.sepsis.org/about/our-mission/.

Vendor Tools

ABOUT: There is an array of vendors that are contracted by hospitals to manage survey data, sample measure populations, submit abstracted data, and a variety of other services. I mention these vendor tools because many of them provide excellent continuing education sources and employ a panel of experts to stay current on regulations. Vendor tool contractors can be an excellent partner in solving problems and understanding processes.

PROS: Usually, a personal contact is provided so that clients can reach out directly with questions.

CONS: Vendors are a business with business interests, so if a QI project is going to increase the vendor's time or expense, it may result in a dead end. Changing vendor tools is also a big headache, so it is hard to achieve results when problems are noted in their services.

Quality Improvement Organizations (QIOs)

ABOUT: QIOs are part of the federal Health and Human Services National Quality Strategy to improve the quality and efficiency of care for Medicare patients. QIOs are also a requirement under the Social Security Act to further the quality of care for Medicare beneficiaries. These QIOs also review violations of the Emergency Medical Treatment and Labor Act (EMTALA) which requires timely stabilization of ED patients. A directory of QIOs is available online, and there will typically be a QIO available for each specific region.[18]

PROS: QIOs can provide more specific data comparing a facility to the regional and national averages. The experts available at QIOs are often able to assist with CMS-related quality reporting questions (such as CMS CDAC Validation appeals). As a Medicare-driven program,

---

18   The Centers for Medicare & Medicaid Services (n.d.). Quality Improvement Organizations. Retrieved March 18, 2022, from https://www.cms.gov/Medicare/Quality-Initiatives-Patient-Assessment-Instruments/QualityImprovementOrgs.

the selected projects are relevant to local facilities and mindful of the bottom line.

CONS: It can be confusing to use the data comparison reports if facility data does not appear to match the data provided by the QIO. Since these organizations are quite large, it can be difficult to obtain individualized feedback to discuss the reports provided by the QIO, and it may take some extra time and work to track down and develop a good relationship with a regional QIO contact for each quality topic.

Chapter 5
Abstraction & Public Reporting

While there truly are many resources available for a successful training experience, it is not uncommon for clever abstractors to be completely unaware of those resources. Abstraction training is often conducted as a quick overview and then "goodbye and good luck." Sometimes, the location of the most recent specifications manual is dependent on a secondary source, and supplemental materials are not discovered for years. It is not a lack of diligence, as many abstractors will search for resources and ask for help, but for the uninitiated, the jargon is unique, and it's difficult to even know how to search for more information. Sometimes the specifications manual for a new registry program is hidden behind a paywall, and accurate training and preparation cannot be done until the contracts are signed. For that matter, in many facilities, it can be hard to find experienced people to ask. Nationally, we are experiencing a labor shortage and healthcare is one of the chief areas of need, so it is not surprising that so many Quality Improvement (QI) professionals need a solid guide to what is expected for a healthy data abstraction program.[1]

Oversight & Reporting Organizations: An Overview

Where would we be without data? Our analysts would have nothing

---

1   American Hospital Association (Nov. 1, 2021). Fact Sheet: Strengthening the Health Care Workforce. Retrieved on March 18, 2022, from https://www.aha.org/fact-sheets/2021-05-26-fact-sheet-strenghtening-health-care-workforce.

to analyze, and our leaders would be forced to lead blindly. Despite the importance of the data provided through abstraction, abstractors still face a veritable support desert when it comes to professional development. To help traverse that desert, this chapter includes information on the abstraction process, including how and why measures are selected, details on retrospective and concurrent abstraction (including where to find each specifications manual), Inter-Rater Reliability (IRR) methods and scoring, and CDAC Validation. But before launching into the details of measure-sample methodology, it would be best to know why it exists in the first place. To answer this question, we must take a look at the key players in healthcare oversight.

Meet the Acronyms:

HHS, CDC, CMS, TJC, DNV, AHA, and Others

Most healthcare professionals are familiar with at least some of these organizational acronyms, but it may be more difficult to describe the various roles of these different organizations, their purpose, the resources they offer, and what they expect from us. So, let's start unpacking who these healthcare acronyms are:

Institutional-Assessment Acronyms

HHS

Each stage of government has a health department: federal, state, and even county. For example, at the federal level, the U.S. Department of Health and Human Services (HHS) exists to improve the health of the nation through research and services.[2] The Health Services Department at the state level has a similar focus with additional details for the specific needs of the state: In Florida, information is provided for citizens to prepare for hurricanes and find available shelters, whereas

---

2　Department of Health and Human Services. (n.d.). About HHS. Retrieved Oct. 25, 2022, from https://www.hhs.gov/about/index.html.

in Montana, information on bear attack prevention is readily available. Then our County Health Departments collect and report health statistics or provide direct services to the community, depending on the priorities and needs of the population. Overall, I would say the historic purpose of health departments at all levels is to reduce risk and improve resiliency in the governed population.

CDC

In addition, the Center for Disease Control and Prevention (CDC) collects data primarily from public health officials and the facility Infection Preventionist related to infectious disease and hospital-acquired infections. The CDC provides guidance to healthcare professionals on disease management, supports testing services, and responds to public health hazards.[3] The QI professional may be involved in hospital-acquired infection surveillance and carrying out a robust infection prevention training program as these initiatives are essential for delivering quality care and patient safety. The collaboration between Infection Prevention and the Quality Department varies widely by the facility, however.

CMS

One of the major players in quality improvement is the Center for Medicare and Medicaid Services (CMS), a federal provider of health insurance for at-risk populations such as the elderly or children living in poverty. CMS is managed by the Department of Health and Human Services (HHS) and provides guidance on healthcare regulations to improve care and make it cost-effective.[4] CMS provides standards for specific diagnoses, such as heart failure or sepsis, across different stages of care such as inpatient hospitalization or home health. Facilities that

---

3   The Center for Disease Control (n.d.). History. Retrieved Oct. 25, 2022, from https://www.cdc.gov/about/history/index.html.

4   The Centers for Medicare & Medicaid Services (n.d.) About CMS. Retrieved Oct. 25, 2022, from https://www.cms.gov/About-CMS.

participate in CMS insurance programs endeavor to meet the quality standards published by CMS because CMS will dock a percentage of payments for healthcare services and issue fines if standards are not met. Some of those penalties result in daily fines that will continue until the hospital is compliant. Healthcare facilities lose billions of dollars to CMS fines every year.

TJC

The Joint Commission (TJC) also provides quality measures for hospitals to abstract and report, but the purpose of the organization is unique: The Joint Commission is a not-for-profit global organization that provides direct surveys of hospital safety for accreditation purposes, as well as guidelines and educational support in patient safety and quality.[5] Where CMS identifies opportunities for improvement and affordability as a federal insurance payor, hospitals actually pay TJC to provide standards for error reduction, prevention of patient harm, and quality measures for clinical performance. Both organizations require the submission of data based on the type and scope of services provided by a hospital. They have their own measures and specifications manuals, and they are submitted separately—but thankfully, TJC works with CMS to prevent duplication.

It is important for the QI professional to take time to become aware of which measures belong to CMS and which ones belong to TJC so that abstraction questions can be answered quickly. Knowing the location of these resources will save significant time. This information can easily be captured with a brief "cheat sheet" to list the applicable measures under the correct organization so that the abstraction team knows where to look for additional details without needing to conduct a blind internet search.

---

5   The Joint Commission (2022). Who We Are. Retrieved on Aug 10, 2022, from https://www.jointcommission.org/who-we-are/facts-about-the-joint-commission/.

DNV

Another organization that provides direct hospital surveys would be Det Norske Veritas (DNV), an international for-profit organization based in Norway that focuses on risk management to "safeguard life, property and the environment."[6] DNV also conducts research and development in other corporate sectors, but for the healthcare QI professional, interaction would focus on hospital survey readiness, results, and accreditation. DNV is not as common as TJC in the United States, but its popularity is increasing, and many hospitals employ both organizations to assess and certify the safety of their care.

Diagnosis-Specific Acronyms

The purpose of a third-party assessment of patient quality, safety and risk is that bias regarding problems can be reduced or removed. The third-party assessment can also ideally help management identify critical improvement projects and enhance the facility's reputation in the community by marketing their accreditation achievements. For a bit more information on hospital surveys and accreditation, see the **Data Analysis** chapter with the section on Survey Data.

Several other organizations help hospitals market their certification achievements, but instead of accrediting the entire facility, these certifications are for effective care of a specific patient diagnosis. There may be a fee to participate and many of the programs are entirely voluntary, so programs can vary based on facility characteristics, interests, and services. However, some examples of key players include:

AHA

The American Heart Association (AHA) has programs for data collection and research to guide hospital programs in heart disease and

---

6   Det Norske Veritas (n.d.). About. Retrieved Oct. 28, 2022, from https://www.dnv.com/about/index.html

stroke to reduce illness and death from these diseases.[7]

NCI

The National Cancer Institute (NCI) is led by the National Institutes of Health (NIH) to collect cancer statistics in an effort to reduce the cancer burden in the U.S. population.[8]

TRAUMA REGISTRY

The Trauma Registry is a mandatory report on trauma care for specific types of injury at trauma-certified facilities to help legislators analyze the trauma care system.[9]

There are many other important organizations that track separate aspects of patient care, including the security of patient data, or special requirements related to Indian Health Services (IHS) for delivering care to members of federally recognized tribes, for example. It is critical for the QI professional to ask questions about mandatory and voluntary participation in programs, including an assessment of whether new certifications should be sought in areas of growth so that best practices are maintained. Facilities are often asked to self-select which measures they will participate in based on their size and the services delivered.

Once the measures are selected, the next task is to collect and submit abstracted data in a timely manner.

7　American Heart Institute (n.d.). About us. Retrieved Oct. 28, 2022, from https://www.heart.org/about-us.

8　National Cancer Institute (n.d.). About NCI. Retrieved Oct. 28, 2022, from https://www.cacner.gov/about-nci/overview.

9　Texas Health and Human Services (n.d.). Texas EMS & Trauma Registries – Frequently Asked Questions. Retrieved Oct. 28, 2022, from https://www.dshs.texas.gov/injury/registry/faq.aspx.

What is Abstraction?

Clinical Data Abstraction is gathering information from the medical record about a specific patient encounter to answer questions about quality. Many quality measures are manually abstracted by clinical staff called abstractors, and some abstractors also analyze the data or manage programs in the facility. However, some measures are automated using data crawlers to pull data from pre-defined fields, such as the electronic Clinical Quality Measures (eCQMs) submitted annually to CMS and TJC. Abstraction may occur retrospectively (looking at a past visit record) or concurrently (looking at a current visit record), which is discussed in more detail below.

TECH TIP: AI

An emerging abstraction option is the use of artificial intelligence (AI) to find relevant data in the medical record using Natural Language Processing (NLP) and Machine Learning (ML).

AI tries to understand context and meaning based on commands or specifications rather than reviewing labelled, predefined data fields. AI is now able to find instances of infection and complete registry abstraction with guidance from a human abstractor.

However, many AI tools tend to "hallucinate" and invent data out of thin air, as they use external sources and predictive logic to guess what the next desired outcome should be. In one demonstration I saw an AI system analyze a table with two data points, "estimate" the results, and get the numbers wildly wrong. It is currently not recommended for any facility or organization to use AI for analyzing or abstracting healthcare data without human guidance.

All About Quality Measures

One of the top priorities of Quality Improvement departments is the accurate and timely submission of performance data, but how are these quality measures selected? Each oversight organization has its own method of determining priorities, setting standards, and selecting quality measures. We will take a closer look at CMS and TJC because most QI professionals will work with these measures at some point.

The Affordable Care Act of 2010 (ACA) required CMS to implement Value-Based Purchasing, where healthcare would be reimbursed according to quality (performance) rather than quantity. So CMS payment for healthcare services are based on value rather than volume in an effort to improve quality and safety and reduce cost burdens to the federal government. In order to define how quality and safety should determine that value, the Core Quality Measures Collaborative (CQMC) reviews and prioritizes the most useful, feasible, evidence-based quality measures for the coming fiscal year. The CQMC is hosted by the National Quality Forum (NQF) and includes clinical members, CMS representatives, and professionals from America's Health Insurance Providers (AHIP). Regarding performance pay, facilities that perform poorly on measures in 2022 would have their financial reimbursement from Medicare reduced in 2024 (one fiscal year after the conclusion of the performance year). At most facilities, CMS is the majority payor source representing more patient accounts than private insurance and uninsured sources combined, so the potential for a payment reduction is something that the entire leadership team is interested in avoiding. Likewise, facilities that receive higher payments from CMS may be able to purchase new equipment or improve staffing ratios that could improve patient treatment options for the next fiscal year, for example.[10]

---

10   The Centers for Medicare and Medicaid Services (2022). "Core Measures." Quality Measures. Retrieved March 17, 2022, from https://www.cms.gov/Medicare/Quality-Initiatives-Patient-Assessment-Instruments/QualityMeasures/Core-Measures.

CMS Core Measures are selected when the clinical outcome is so positive that it is reasonable to expect every patient with a specific illness will have an improved outcome if they receive the evidence-based treatment protocol. One of the original core measures, for example, was the timely administration of aspirin to a patient experiencing a myocardial infarct (a.k.a. a "heart attack"), because "patient outcomes were significantly improved by timely aspirin administration, and cost burdens increased for patients who did not receive timely aspirin and experienced poor outcomes."[11]

TJC has a similar process of collaborating with a variety of stakeholders, including CMS, to determine their clinical quality measure selections each year. At TJC, measures that are feasible to monitor and have evidence of improved patient outcomes without significant adverse effects are called "accountability measures" and will affect pay-for-performance, public reporting, or accreditation in some way.[12]

Retrospective Abstraction

Mandatory abstraction occurs retrospectively, which means it is a chart review that occurs after the patient has discharged and the final coding is complete. This means that retrospective abstraction occurs when changes to patient care generally cannot be made. However, many professionals ask if they are allowed to make late entries to the retrospective documentation. The intent of abstraction is to use only documentation that was part of the medical record during the encounter, but there are times when a provider addendum or late entry is added after discharge to correct a documentation omission or to

11   Wright, R. S., et al (May 2011). 2011 ACCF/AHA Focused Update of the Guidelines for the Management of Patient With Unstable Angina/Non-ST-Elevation Myocardial Infarction (Updating the 2007 Guideline). *J Am Coll Cardiol, 57* (19): 1920-59. https://www.jacc.org/doi/abs/10.1016/j.jacc.2011.02.009.

12   The Joint Commission (2022). Measures. Retrieved on March 17, 2022, from https://www.jointcommission.org/measurement/measures/.

clarify ambiguous or non-specific documentation. This late entry or addendum can only be used in abstraction if it is documented within 30 days of discharge based on rules for timely medical record completion published by CMS; these late entries and addendums must follow ethical guidelines, as well as legal guidelines outlined in the Code of Federal Regulations for medical record services.[13] As long as the purpose of the late entry is to clarify and improve documentation (and not to improve scores), an abstractor who completes their review in a timely manner may submit a query to the physician about the rationale behind care decisions, and improvements to the documentation may consequently improve abstraction accuracy. For example, a patient with a massive GI bleed and hemorrhagic shock may have no documentation of a reason to hold the anticoagulant at discharge for atrial fibrillation, but a query to the physician within 30 days of discharge may ask them to explain why the medication was held. If the physician documents that the patient's hemorrhage was the reason for holding the medication, it would clarify the care decisions that were made and answer a required abstraction query that was previously unable to determine (UTD).

Each retrospective measure includes a process document with a measure algorithm to describe how to review the medical chart step-by-step for that specific measure. The process document is found in the specifications manual, which is the complete guide to abstraction for the measure. Any "cheat sheets" or unofficial guidance used must not contradict the specifications manual.

Common Manuals

CMS

CMS manuals can be found at https://qualitynet.cms.gov/. Select

---

13   The Code of Federal Regulations (2022). "Medicare Conditions of Participation: Medical Record Services." National Archives, 42 C.F.R. § 482.24 C(4)(viii). Retrieved March 18, 2022, from https://www.ecfr.gov/current/title-42/chapter-IV/subchapter-G/part-482.

"Hospital-Inpatient," "Hospital-Outpatient," or "Inpatient Psychiatric Facilities," and the page will open with the respective specifications manual links. There is an alphabetical data dictionary in the list of documents, and it is searchable (use the Command-F "Fast Find" feature). There is also a Question & Answer Tool for requesting clarification to interpret the manual accurately (https://cmsqualitysupport. servicenowservices.com/qnet_qa). Anyone can submit a question and responses are typically emailed. There is also a library of Frequently Asked Questions (FAQs) about the measures.

TJC

Manuals for all specifications, including eCQMs can be found at https://www.jointcommission.org/measurement/specification-manuals/. However, a quick link to the manually abstracted measures would be https://manual.jointcommission.org/. Select the manual by the patient's discharge date. There is an alphabetical data dictionary at the bottom of the list of measures and the measure documents are searchable (use the Command-F "Fast Find" feature). There is also a Question & Answer Tool to clarify and interpret the specifications (https://manual.jointcommission.org/Home/MyQuestions).

AHA

Get With the Guidelines (GWTG) programs: The manual can be found at: https://www.heart.org/en/professional/quality-improvement/. Scroll down and select the program to find fact sheets, or login to the abstraction tool at https://aha.infosarioregistry.com/login and click on "Library" to find the current specification guidelines. The "Contact" link allows us to send questions about interpreting the specifications to the assigned AHA contact for each region.

Algorithms

Within the measure algorithm, the first abstraction questions typically ask whether the patient visit belongs in the population or whether exclusions apply (demographics, comfort care, etc.). Abstracting an exclusion will remove the patient from the sample and additional cases will be sampled to meet the sampling requirements.

See *Figure 5.1A* for an example of the population algorithm from the specifications manual for the Joint Commission's Perinatal Care - Exclusive Breast Milk Feeding measure (PC-05).[14]

The algorithm shows that only patients born alive with a specified length of stay and diagnosis code will be included in the population to screen for breastfeeding. While the algorithm looks confusing, most vendor tools manage the population sampling automatically for the abstractor, so it is usually just a matter of verifying that the correct list of diagnosis codes and visit dates are entered into the vendor tool.

Once a patient is determined to be part of the measure population, the actual clinical care questions begin and will result in a pass or fail score. (see *Figure 5.1B*)

The algorithm shows that answering "Yes" to the query "Admission to NICU" would result in "B - Not in Measure Population." In other words, if the baby was critically ill, TJC will not hold hospitals accountable for successful breastfeeding. Likewise, if the baby is not term (at least 37 weeks gestation at birth), the measure will result in "B - Not in Measure Population," and TJC accepts that there was at least a valid clinical reason for other feeding choices. The "B - Not in Measure Population" result is called the category assignment, and each case has a category assignment by the time abstraction is completed. For this example, the category assignments are listed below with explanations:

- X = Case will be rejected (usually due to incomplete answers). This is bad because it would result in a failed submission to CMS. Any incomplete cases should be abstracted and resolved prior to submission to CMS.

14   The Joint Commission (2022). Perinatal Care - Exclusive Breast Milk Feeding (PC-05) Measure Algorithm. *Specifications Manual for Joint Commission National Quality Measures* (v2022B1). Retrieved Oct. 25, 2022, from https://manual.jointcommission.org/releases/TJC2022B1/MIF0170.html.

FIG 5.1A
JOINT COMMISSION'S PERINATAL CARE - EXCLUSIVE BREAST MILK FEEDING MEASURE (PC-05)

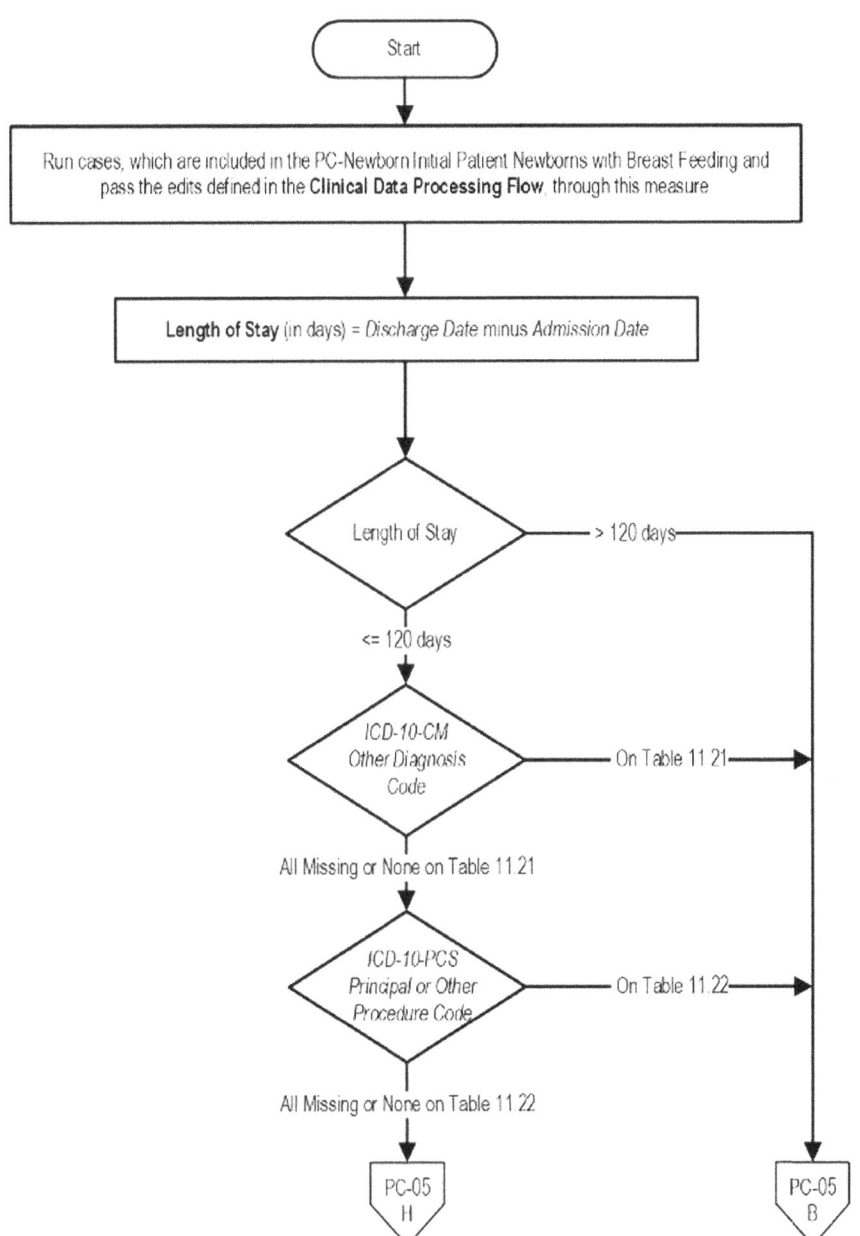

FIG 5.1B
JOINT COMMISSION'S PERINATAL CARE - EXCLUSIVE
BREAST MILK FEEDING MEASURE (PC-05 CONT.)

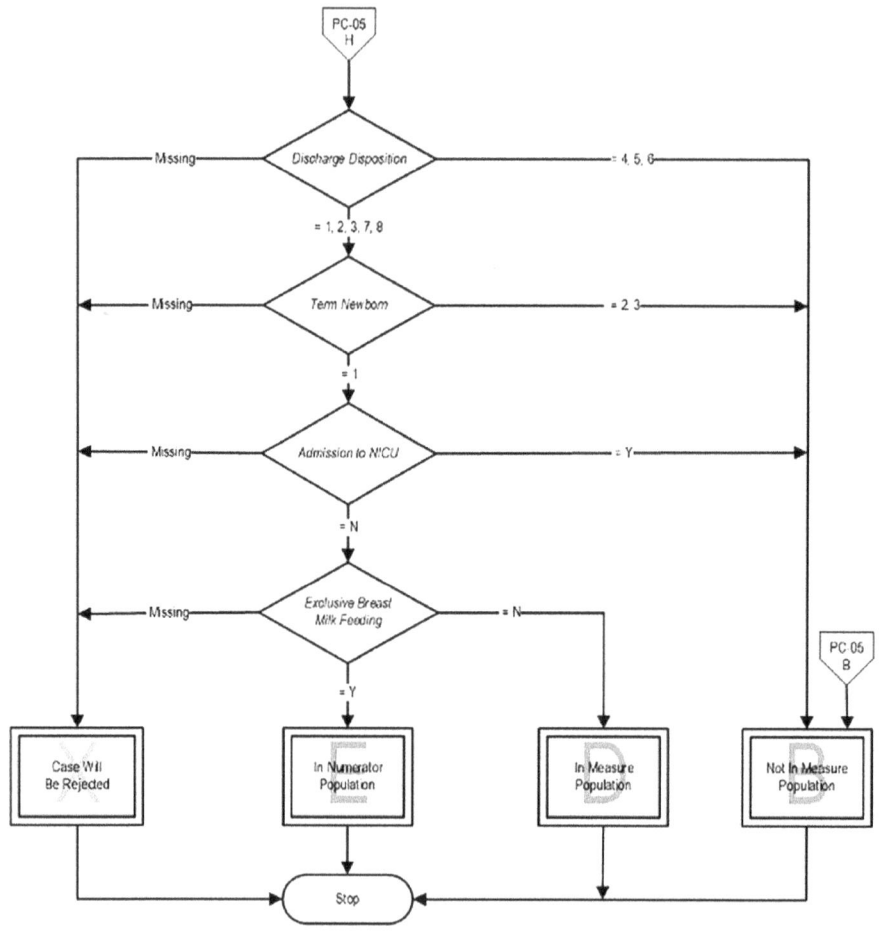

- E = Case is included and passes the quality measure queries. This is good news!

- D = Case is included in the population but fails the quality measure guidelines. Ah, sadness. These are the cases to study for process improvement so that future cases will not fail. A failure is also optimistically called an "opportunity for improvement," or an "OFI" by QI professionals.

- B = Case is excluded from measure population based on abstracted answers. Basically, this means the case was initially in the population based on coding and length of stay, but then maybe the patient went to NICU for a short time and that abstracted answer excludes the case. If there are lots of excluded cases, the sample may need to be corrected to include enough cases to meet CMS sampling requirements.

It's important to study the exact algorithm for each specific measure because some category assignments are reversed: Where the exclusive breastfeeding measure is asking "was the best, evidence-based outcome achieved?" there are other measures asking, "did the patient experience the worst outcome?" An example of this type of measure is the AHA's Hemorrhagic Stroke question about whether a bleed occurred after thrombolytic treatment. A bleed after treatment would be a bad outcome for the patient, so the category assignment is reversed. Instead of answering "Yes, a good thing happened" the measure answers, "Yes, a bad thing happened." So in the bleeding question, a positive "E" category assignment would be considered a bad thing, but a category assignment of "D" is passing (the exact reverse of most measures). The good news is that most vendor tools offer a report that shows color-coding for the category assignment outcome (green for passing, red for failures, and some other demure color to indicate an exclusion).

Some quality topics, like the stroke treatment measures, are divided into multiple measures where a patient encounter could potentially have multiple failures. Some contain "parent" questions that will open dependent "child" questions such as the AHA's Heart Failure registry, where additional requirements for discharge medications will open when there is evidence of severe left ventricular systolic dysfunction (LVSD). Other topics might be bundled into an all-in-one measure such as sepsis, where there is one measure to capture early recognition and treatment, and a single failure will cause the entire measure to fail.

The specifications manuals are routinely updated and each of the organization websites listed above include an invitation to sign-up for a listserv, and they even have helpful webinars to explain any abstraction updates. It's easy to sign-up to receive these invitations, and I would highly recommend it because updates and changes may alter critical work activities.

Perhaps your work does not require direct abstraction, but you are asked to monitor progress and abstraction results. What do the measure scores mean? When a measure fails, it is called a fallout or, more optimistically, an opportunity for improvement (OFI). Every fallout should be reviewed for accuracy by the abstractor and a program analyst. This may involve an action plan if the facility believes a thorough and immediate correction should be made. Fallout correction plans should be based on the findings of a thorough investigation, and the correction itself should be measurable and specific to the point of failure. For example, if an abstractor is found to be using only a portion of the medical record to abstract and neglecting to review scanned, handwritten notes, the fallout may be a process error rather than a clinical performance error, and an action plan might include education about the CMS guidelines for included documents in measure abstraction, and close monitoring with extra IRR cases over a period of 90 days. Don't worry—IRR is described in the next section.

For developing a corrective plan when clinical performance and patient care is below the standard, please see the **Project Management** chapter.

Inter-Rater Reliability (IRR)

If abstractors were in school, their "grade" would be an IRR match report. In fact, CMS requires several proofs to demonstrate that facilities are abstracting their charts accurately, and not just fudging the numbers to get the full Medicare reimbursement. One of these requirements is called **Inter-Rater Reliability**, which occurs when a retrospective abstraction is complete. IRR is the gold standard of abstraction performance, and it is intended to show the reliability of the abstractor's data. Here's how it works: A second abstractor who has no pre-existing knowledge of the patient chart will conduct a **blind abstraction**, not looking at any previous abstraction answers recorded by the first abstractor. If they match perfectly, there is no further work. If they don't match, each mismatch needs to be reviewed. During review, either the original or the IRR abstractor is found to be inaccurate, and the result is recorded. These results are then used for performance review and educational planning. IRR is usually conducted each quarter at a minimum (though it can be done more frequently), and the results are finalized and shared with leadership, until it is eventually reported to CMS where the score affects annual payments.

The IRR results include two types of scoring. There is a Data Element Agreement Rate (DEAR), which looks at every element (or question) in the abstraction. The DEAR is helpful to determine an abstractor's knowledge of the elements, overall performance, and for identifying knowledge gaps on the team. The second score is a Category Assignment Agreement Rate (CAAR) which looks at the measure outcome and is expressed as a percentage match rate. If the original category assignment was "E" and the IRR category assignment was "E," then the CAAR matches (even if there are individual elements that do not match perfectly). Only the CAAR score is reported to CMS. When the CAAR score is available, most facilities require a corrective action plan for a quarterly CAAR of less than 90% per measure, and some may require a higher threshold.

The accuracy of retrospective data abstraction is critical because it informs policy and program decisions, but clearly the individual patient experience cannot be altered after discharge: No one can go back in time to a patient's inpatient admission date and administer an aspirin or apply venous thromboembolism (VTE) prophylaxis. Because of this time limitation, some facilities request concurrent abstraction to allow QI professionals to keep tabs on current projects in real-time.

Concurrent Abstraction

Sometimes it can be frustrating to see poor scores from retrospective abstraction and wish that those patients could have had a better experience. Other times, the Quality Department may be suspicious that hospital staff are still not clear on what they need to do to fulfill measure requirements. In this case, it is ideal to have real-time practice in improving the patient's care rather than wish that the hospital had a time machine. And it would be even better if QI could deliver on-the-spot education for staff who are struggling to apply the measure, right?

This is where concurrent abstraction shines. It is a fancy name, but it is a simple concept. When you find a measure that needs real-time help with performance issues, it is a good time to start compiling patient lists on a daily basis and checking to see that measure requirements are getting done in a timely manner. Once these patients are identified, discussions can occur with the patient's provider in real time to uncover barriers and opportunities.

That sounds wonderful from a program management perspective, but it must be said that concurrent abstraction is a beastly time burden for QI staff. Concurrent abstraction is the most common task to hand off to clinical staff who are on light duty from the nursing unit (an entry point for many quality professionals), and it is stressful to review holiday and weekend coverage when daily monitoring is deemed necessary. So take caution in selecting a measure for concurrent abstraction, and make sure that it is a priority from both a reporting and leadership standpoint.

Assuming that leadership is invested, and reporting agencies believe the measure is critical, how would a QI professional actually find those patients when there is no diagnosis code on arrival? Remember that coding occurs after discharge, and the rapid diagnoses written into the Emergency Department (ED) visit can be quite vague, like "cough, weakness." So how can the patient census be filtered to only pull patients with a specific diagnosis? In retrospective abstraction, the vendor tool pulls relevant patients based on their discharge coding. However, when the patient has not discharged, it is definitely more difficult to identify which patients need review and which ones are not applicable. I personally recall many IT tickets and phone calls waiting for someone to explain how this might be done for a particular patient population, and it often required some type of new access to my IT profile that would allow me to view the current ED Census, for example. Below are a couple of examples to provide ideas for your program, but do not be afraid to reach out for help from the IT department if you are struggling to get access to a relevant resource:

- The SEP-1 measure required early recognition and treatment within three hours, so post-discharge review was not sufficient. A sepsis screening was launched by the Informatics Department, however, and an IT analyst was able to provide access to the ED Census to review positive sepsis screenings. Additional access to positive screening reports were also provided, and we initiated a concurrent review process for sepsis based on positive nurse sepsis screenings, ED admission diagnoses, and code sepsis alerts called in the ED and duplicated on the sepsis coordinator's pager. Daily compliance scores were provided in leadership board meetings each morning.

- Both the stroke registry and stroke core measure required timely recognition and treatment of stroke patients. All stroke patients except an occasional outlier were admitted through the ED, so a Code Stroke Alert was initiated most of the time. This alert was called overhead and submitted to the stroke coordinator's pager. A process of "CT Scan First" was initiated with EMS stroke alert patients so that patients would go to radiology on arrival, rather than an ED bed. The radiology department would then call a critical value to the ED when a stroke was possible from the scan. The list of stroke alerts were then reviewed each day to ensure that all quality measures were in place from day one through discharge. Performance was reviewed with the chief neurologist on a weekly basis.

- The venous thromboembolism (VTE) measure to prevent blood clots in hospital patients required the initiation of prophylaxis within one day of the inpatient admission. Since this measure included the entire adult inpatient population, a list of inpatient admissions (today minus one day) would be printed and reviewed for prophylaxis. A warfarin report was also provided by pharmacy for monitoring of the warfarin quality measures, and reminders were sent to the charge nurse in case the patient should discharge. Patients missing VTE prophylaxis were reported daily in leadership board meetings to allow the charge nurse to ask questions about unique situations, such as intubated amputees.

These examples show how concurrent review can be used to improve a critical program, but it also shows the complexity of this type of project: multi-level leadership involvement, changes to medical record screenings and security access, daily tallies on performance, and the potential of a pager going off in the middle of the night to report a positive alert can be a formidable project. It helps to plan ahead for a "launch date" and trial the surveillance process. Whatever method is chosen, it will undoubtedly have imperfections, and changes may or may not be possible, but it is always worth asking. Any concurrent review should be part of a larger program management plan, and support should be provided to accomplish such an ambitious task.

Sampling & Submission

We have discussed a great deal about the purpose and process of abstraction. Let's take a step back now for some high-level details on how a quality manager would determine which measures are required, how many patients need to be abstracted, and where to submit the abstraction.

Earlier in the chapter, the CMS specifications manual landing page was shared (https://qualitynet.cms.gov/). From this page, if you click on a category (Hospitals-Inpatient) and click on the Data Management tab, you will find information on the CMS Abstraction & Reporting Tool (CART). The direct website for Inpatient Data Management is https://qualitynet.cms.gov/inpatient/data-management and this site also includes information on data submission, including formatting and key deadlines. Further, this section of the site explains Data Validation ("CDAC"), which we will discuss near the end of this chapter.

The CART site is where records are submitted electronically to the national warehouse, and clicking into the CART page and selecting the CART Resources tab will take you to a training page. The training page has tips on getting started with the application itself, as well as training modules on how to use it correctly (https://qualitynet.cms.gov/inpatient/data-management/cart/resources#tab2). The CART page is also where the quality manager would attest to the completeness of data and provide security clearance for third party vendor tools if they will be submitting data on behalf of the facility.

The CART page is a key resource for successful submission of manually abstracted measures as well as approval of submission for electronic measures (eCQMs). But the other resource to consider is the specifications manuals, where population and sampling requirements are discussed for each measure. Hospitals are not required to sample, which means they may submit a 100% sample of eligible patient charts, but that is probably more time-consuming and expensive than figuring out the sample methodology. Most facilities will find the minimum sample required by the specifications manual based on the number of patients, beds, or births at their facility, and then it is wise to round up with a comfortable margin to cover any charts excluded during abstraction. The folks at CMS know their statistics quite well, and in my experience, 100% sampling was not particularly beneficial because the required sample size provides an accurate picture of care performance. Also, since the sample itself is based on diagnosis codes, each update to the manual's coding inclusion and exclusion list will mean extra reviews at the time of the change to ensure that the correct cases are getting picked up in the sampling process.

Most facilities use third party vendor tools for submission of data to CMS, but the facility still needs to provide guidelines to the vendor on sample methodology and preferences. An important activity for collaboration is the **normalization** of data, which is where additional patient charts are pulled into the sample if a large enough number of patients were excluded during abstraction. Normalization adjustments can be reduced by including a larger margin above the required sample size.

For example, if the Outpatient Emergency Department Throughput (OP-ED) sample includes several patients who visited the ED for some sort of follow-up care—like picking up a prescription for an antibiotic based on culture results or the removal of stitches—those patients would be removed during abstraction from the sample because they did not see a physician for a medical screening exam (MSE). Without seeing the physician for an assessment in the ED, there is no billing for an Outpatient Evaluation and Management (E/M) Code, and E/M Codes of "none available" are automatically excluded from the sample when selected by the abstractor in the vendor tool. The same process occurs for Inpatient Sepsis every time a patient is marked "No" for severe sepsis.

The vendor tool will typically include a display of the number of sampled patients with completed abstractions. This display should be reviewed routinely for abstraction progress as well as the potential need for sample size adjustments through normalization. Given the need for sample size fulfillment, it is logical to complete abstraction cases early, and the deadline for routine normalization should be carefully determined with the vendor tool to ensure that there is time to abstract any freshly sampled cases. If abstraction is backlogged and normalization throws a new case load into the mix, there could be significant stress for the abstraction team to meet mandatory reporting deadlines.

Another reason for checking the sample early is to look for errors. For example, January cases are prone to errors because updates in coding often occur in January, and abstractors are also more prone to human error as they may enter the previous year in the date entries due to habit. These errors, along with any missing data, need to be resolved prior to submission to CMS. Error resolution should be done by the facility prior to the final submission trial. If it is not done in advance, the errors will still be reported at the last minute by the vendor tool as barriers to timely submission, and that would induce a stressful day for the whole department. Thankfully, the vendor tool includes a display of errors by type (missing data, invalid entry, etc.), and representatives from the vendor tool company are usually more than willing to show analysts where to look for the errors in their system and how to resolve them.

Finally, when the quarter is completely abstracted, normalized, and all errors are resolved, the vendor tool will do a test submission. Every facility does this test submission to make sure that there is time to resolve problems, because CMS makes almost no exceptions for late or missing entries (unless they have declared an official emergency). If there are any unexpected issues during the test submission, the vendor will let the facility know so that corrections can be made immediately, and the submission will be re-tested prior to the final submission date posted by CMS.

Since there is quite a bit of collaboration with medical records and the vendor tool, it is important to communicate about the process. It is completely acceptable to send a check-in email to the vendor tool letting them know when abstraction is complete and to please let you know if there are any issues noted. Your contact at the vendor tool will also be able to communicate about their deadlines—likely for the entire year ahead—for test submissions and error audits. They can help with technical difficulties, coding updates, error review, and questions about CMS and TJC. Additionally, many vendor tools offer educational webinars or newsletters about abstraction changes and announcements, and these are a valuable resource for the QI professional.

While this section focused on mandatory CMS submission, the

process for mandatory TJC submission is quite similar: Submission of the perinatal measures, for example, is typically managed by the same vendor tool and would follow a quarterly schedule posted on TJC's website. All errors and incomplete cases should be reviewed prior to the submission deadline.

The mandatory submission of quarterly trauma data to the national trauma registry is usually managed at the state level through the department of health, and the cancer and tumor registries have their own pathway to submission to the federal registries. The infection preventionist, meanwhile, will have a different federal submission pathway for infection reporting.

For voluntary abstraction programs such as the AHA's Get With The Guidelines (GWTG) programs for stroke or heart disease, the deadlines may be as infrequent as an annual submission. However, the burden of abstraction is heavier and more detailed than many of the CMS/TJC required abstractions. For these measures, your facility will be assigned to a professional contact within the organization who can answer questions about interpreting the specifications manual, the status of your facility towards earning awards, and opportunities for education and performance improvement. It is wise to schedule regular meetings with your contact and prepare an agenda for the meeting. Your contact will be ready to share your progress reports toward the awards in question, but it is the QI professional's responsibility to take advantage of the meeting by writing down questions that refer to the manual, or to ask about specific problems. If you are starting a new program, they may connect you with a mentor who is experienced and that is an excellent opportunity to look at examples in a live environment and ask about problem areas or any area that is confusing to the abstraction team.

It is critical that the QI manager is aware of each program with its unique guidelines, submission deadlines, and auditing practices, to ensure that facility performance is measured in a timely manner, and that decisions can be made when there is still time to make adjustments in the relevant program. For this reason, it is wise to set up recurring meetings with abstraction staff and vendor tool contacts to ensure that all requirements for submission are met in a timely manner for each relevant program.

CDAC Validation

One of the mysteries of quality reporting is the Clinical Data Abstraction Center (CDAC) Validation process. CDAC carries a heavy financial weight for hospitals, and the mere mention of the term can make experienced QI professionals shiver with fear. I honestly thought there must be some sort of on-site torture involved based on the way people responded to the term. In truth, CDAC is an audit of hospital abstraction that is similar to Inter Rater Reliability (IRR), yet it can feel more like an IRS audit for many QI professionals. And it is just as impactful: Failing validation can result in a reduction in CMS reimbursement across the board. This means that low scores on CDAC will prompt a visit from the CFO to your office (and it won't be a pleasant chat with coffee). One way to alleviate stress during CDAC Validation is to become familiar with the process and have an awareness of potential pitfalls, which we will discuss shortly. At this point, I have completed dozens of rounds of CDAC Validation, and I no longer break out in a sweat when I see my facility's name on the validation list, so let's start at the beginning and demystify this whole validation process.

So, what is CDAC? It is basically quality control by CMS to ensure that abstraction data is accurate—like an IRR audit by CMS experts. They want to make sure that abstractors understand the specifications and are following them consistently, so they collect a random sample of all facilities nation-wide and pull a sample of the submitted charts for review. An expert abstractor at CMS reviews inpatient/outpatient charts that were previously sampled and submitted for core measures for each of those facilities. The expert at CMS abstracts the patient charts blindly according to CMS specifications, and then compares their expert abstraction against the submitted hospital abstraction. The hospital's abstraction is scored based on how closely their answers match the expert, and educational comments are provided by the expert to help the facility improve their knowledge of the measure. If a passing rate is not achieved, the CDAC audit is automatically repeated the following year with financial consequences for not passing, meaning failing CDAC will cost your facility significant income, and the auditing will continue until the accuracy threshold is met.

Because of the financial impact, CDAC submission can be a stressful time with added scrutiny from administration. If the submitted records have significant abstraction errors, a hospital will not receive full reimbursement from CMS for the future fiscal year selected. CMS states that hospitals that fail CDAC will receive "their annual market basket update with a reduction by one-fourth of the applicable market basket update."[15] One-fourth or 25% is a very large number when it comes to reimbursement. Needless to say, CDAC Validation is a high priority for every Quality Department. The following section describes where to find information from CMS, what is expected of the Quality Department during CDAC, what the scores mean, and some potential resources in case something goes wrong.

Where can a QI professional find out whether their facility is on CDAC Validation this year? CMS publishes a list on their website of the facilities that will be audited for inpatient and outpatient abstraction each year.[16] CMS also sends a request by mail, and they notify hospital leadership by email. If contact information is not updated with CMS and mail is "undeliverable," CMS will research the contacts and request updates to the CMS system.

It is a good idea to look up the facility validation list on the CMS website each year and sign-up for the CMS newsletters to be fully aware

---

15   The Centers for Medicare and Medicaid Services (2022). "Annual Payment Update." Hospital Inpatient Quality Reporting (IQR) Program. Retrieved March 8, 2022, from https://qualitynet.cms.gov/inpatient/iqr/apu. Accessed March 8, 2022.

16   The Centers for Medicare and Medicaid Services (2022). "Data Validation: Resources." Data Management. Retrieved on March 8, 2022, from https://qualitynet. cms.gov/inpatient/data-management/data-validation/resources.

of deadlines for chart submission and CDAC Validation. From the CMS Inpatient or Outpatient homepage, select Data Management > Data Validation to find a variety of resources on CDAC Validation. This same website has information about how to submit patient charts, timelines for review, and information about making an appeal within 30 days, so it is a good page to bookmark in your browser.

What is expected from the Quality Department? Once the validation period begins, the hospital must send a complete copy of the chart electronically according to the instructions on the CMS website. This will require a cooperative effort between the patient records department and the Quality Department, so it is good to reach out to the Health Information Management (HIM) director early on and discuss the process and deadlines for CDAC submission.

It is imperative to review each patient chart prior to sending to CMS for CDAC submission. They should be reviewed in great detail, reviewing each answer and confirming that the source document is in the chart where CMS can find it (the source document is any source used for the original abstraction). For example, if a heart rate of 109 is used for sepsis presentation, the quality professional would review the digital chart and make sure that same heart rate is located in the vital signs documents and is included for CMS to review. If CMS cannot review the heart rate, the abstraction may not match, and the case could fail. Also, be sure to verify which measure is being submitted. For example, if the chart for patient X was initially abstracted for both OP-ED Throughput and OP-Stroke, the CDAC chart request form will show which measure type is requested for CDAC review. Again, CMS urges hospitals to send the complete chart and to verify that there are no missing records.

Keep in mind that the original abstraction was already submitted and processed by CMS, so **no changes should be made to any abstractions** at this point. If a potential mistake is found in the abstraction, it should not be corrected. Rather, the goal of this review is to ensure that nothing is missing from the copied chart.

This may seem obvious, but in my experience, a significant number of facilities fail CDAC Validation each year because an incomplete chart was sent to CMS. The documentation received by CMS is then abstracted, and it cannot match the original abstraction, which utilized a whole and complete patient chart. These facilities could fail CDAC even if their abstraction performance is flawless. And worse, appeals for not checking these details prior to submission are generally rejected unless there is some additional reason for accommodation, and they cannot even be filed until the Validation period is concluded. Additional pages cannot be added after submission, and in the guide to hospitals, it says: "CMS strongly recommends hospitals review and perform quality assurance on the information included within the medical records submitted to the CDAC to assure that all necessary documentation is included." They recommend this review to ensure the chart is complete and also to provide assurance that details such as the date of service, encounter number, and patient identification also match. Suffice it to say, CDAC validation is a good opportunity to consult experienced guidance and check the chart repeatedly for completeness and accuracy in an all-hands-on-deck review.

It is also wise to keep in mind that, due to the financial impact of CDAC Validation scores, the QI professional should be highly cautious about providing any estimate or prediction of results in advance. Analysts in the Quality Department may wish to speculate on pre-submission reviews to guess whether the quarter will pass or fail, but it is impossible to know until the expert reviewer provides educational guidance and scoring of the charts. If a predicted score is shared prior to the official score and is later found to be inaccurate, it can cause a loss of trust at the higher administrative levels of the facility once the official score is available. The best practice is to keep any predictions close-to-cuff and offer clear statements about when an official score can be expected. CMS reports that results are typically available within four months via the secure online portal.

What should be done when scores arrive? When CMS responds, a scoring sheet will be posted online for each chart. Usually, about eight charts are submitted each quarter for either inpatient or outpatient

CDAC, and each chart will be scored separately. The score is based on category assignment (CAAR) rather than each individual abstraction element (DEAR). To find the facility score, divide the number of matches (numerator) by the total possible matches (denominator), and it will result in a percentage score, such as 14 matches out of 16 possible, or 87.5%. The numbers can be confusing, though, as a facility may be audited for infection prevention measures, inpatient and/or outpatient programs, so keeping track of progress can be challenging. Over the course of the audit, I kept a spreadsheet with each quarterly score on the main sheet (both predicted and actual), and maintained separate tabs for each measure where I could document a more detailed case analysis.

How are the scores reported? The different quality programs are calculated separatey by CMS, and the goal is for each program total to achieve a passing score. This means that any abstraction issues with infection prevention reporting would not affect outpatient core measure abstraction scores, for example, because they are counted separately on a pass/fail basis. Let's take a closer look at the program differences:

- The eCQMs are not included in CDAC Validation because they are weighted differently for timely and complete submission instead of accuracy.

- The infection prevention Hospital-Acquired Conditions (HAC) Reduction Program submission is calculated separately for CDAC Validation based on National Healthcare Safety Network (NHSN) reporting accuracy.

- Hospital Inpatient Quality Reporting Program scores are calculated separately from the Outpatient Quality Reporting Program scores. A facility may be selected for one and not the other. If a facility is selected for both, they could fail one and pass the other because they are counted separately.

- Surgical facilities with inpatient visits or transfers may need to watch closely for CDAC Validation, because even if they have one patient in the entire previous year for the core measures sample, they may be audited for accuracy in abstraction of that one case.

Due to these complexities, I recommend counting, re-counting, and reviewing the score sheet and metrics with a knowledgeable peer to prevent miscommunication about scores, especially prior to communicating the numbers to administration.

What is a passing score? Scores are based on the annual total percentage per program. At the time of publication, a passing match rate is an average overall score of 75% over the course of validation. Progress is tracked by adding each quarterly score as the results come in, and it will likely feel a lot like counting points from college exams to figure out how much is needed to pass the final. For example, a score of 64% for first quarter would require a score of at least 86% the next quarter to get back into the passing range of a 75% total. Again, this is a prediction, and discretion is recommended when sharing any predicted scores with administration—but it can potentially provide some peace of mind during the process, as long as it is carefully declared that the numbers are only estimates and not official results. As mentioned, scores cannot be changed but any errors in record completeness or submission process errors could be corrected prior to the next quarter's submission. Those mid-validation process changes can be enough to turn a failing quarterly score into a passing overall score, so it is worth the effort. To this point, CDAC Validation is truly a learning opportunity where a hospital that may otherwise receive no expert feedback on abstraction can receive direct, specific feedback from national experts.

Given the opportunity to see feedback from national experts, the best practice is to review all mismatches and create an action plan for any improvement recommendations, even if a passing score is achieved. I typically use my favorite Root Cause Analysis (RCA) tool because it starts with the question, "what is the normal process?" and this type of investigation offers more insight into the habits of the abstraction team, as well as the clinical team, to find opportunities that may otherwise be missed. Once the root cause is identified (and there may be more than one), the action plan can be created. For more details on how to conduct a Root Cause Analysis for abstraction improvement, please see the **Simple Tools** chapter.

As each quarter is reviewed, parsed, and action plans are created, continue to maintain a running spreadsheet with a tab for each quarter's findings, folders for all CMS reports, and notes on any RCAs or action plans carried out. These notes will be a treasure trove if abstraction methods or CMS responses are questioned in the future, or if any details are requested by administration.

When all is said and done, what should be included in a report to hospital administration? The findings that are gleaned from action plans, and any discoveries or changes that are made, are some of the most useful things to share with administration. Beyond the initial need to assuage financial fears about scoring, the information that is most helpful to administration comes from what the quality team does with CMS feedback. Being able to report a detailed overview of an RCA and case-by-case scores are great ways to show that the quality team is taking CDAC Validation feedback seriously, and that actionable changes are being implemented promptly.

What can be done if the final score does not pass? The first step, again, is a thorough investigation. CMS will likely repeat the CDAC Validation audit the following year, so it is critical to pull all the RCAs together and discuss the results with administration and staff.

- Were there errors in submission?

- Were corrections communicated clearly and understood by the abstraction team?

- Are there ongoing knowledge gaps?

The resolution to these questions could range anywhere from an educational review with CMS, partnering with a regional Quality Improvement Organization (QIO) to improve knowledge gaps, an appeal to CMS due to extraneous problems (such as a natural disaster), an internal disciplinary process, or gathering bids to contract vendor solutions for abstraction so that local staff attention can shift to on-site quality improvement rather than abstraction.

If a hospital has a question or clarification on validation outcomes, the CMS website has information about requesting a Data Validation Educational Review, which must be requested within 30 days of Validation results. In addition, the Quality Improvement Organizations (QIO) are an excellent resource to provide guidance if things go sideways, as they may have educational tips or be able to provide guidance on preparing an appeal to CMS for submission. It is also worth noting that an appeal can only be submitted to CMS if the overall score is below passing. Appeals are not accepted by CMS to discuss whether an 80% could be turned into an 82% for a single quarter, for example. If there are specific questions on how to interpret measure feedback and specifications, there should be details about how to contact the CMS expert reviewer or how to send a clarification question included in the score report. There is also a general Question and Answer section from the QualityNet Support page for measure clarification and support.[17] The CMS Q&A site can be used to search for existing answers (because someone may have already asked the same question) or to ask a measure-specific question in your own words.

It is good to keep in mind that while every facility worries about CDAC Validation, there are so many resources available to make it a positive experience for the team rather than a threatening one. Completing CDAC Validation is also a feather in the cap of anyone working in QI: Once it is over and done, they can serve as an experienced leader who is able to guide others in the process. In closing this topic, if your facility is pulled for CDAC Validation, remember to draw on available resources early on rather than waiting to see the problems, and be sure to check twice before submitting anything to CMS or hospital administration.

---

17   The Centers for Medicare and Medicaid Services (n.d.). QualityNet Support. Retrieved Aug. 9, 2022, from https://qualitynet.cms.gov/support/.

Chapter 6
Interdisciplinary Care

There are definite advantages to working on a team with clearly defined roles, and this section discusses some of the disciplines that work symbiotically with healthcare Quality Improvement (QI). I have included brief descriptions of their unique roles and some potential prospects for collaboration, although there are surely many more opportunities yet to be discovered. The goal of collaboration is to bring the focus of care back to seeing the patient holistically and including the unique perspectives of other healthcare disciplines. Working together, the quality team may "see" the patient more clearly through the additional tools and resources these other disciplines bring to the table.

What is Medical Coding?

As a bedside nurse, I paid no attention to medical coding and lived blissfully unaware of billing and monetary costs of the care I was giving. I never wanted to think of healthcare as a corporate endeavor or distract attention away from the patient. However, in QI it was necessary for me to learn a bit about the coding abstract, which is a legal billing summary that describes care delivered and conditions treated during the encounter. The final coding is done after discharge and is based on physician documentation about treatment delivered and diagnoses that were made during the encounter.

One aspect that directly affects abstraction is whether the coding abstract includes or excludes a diagnosis because it could pull a patient in or out of quality measure samples based on the presence or absence of a code. For example, if a patient is initially suspected for a stroke and the patient history later reveals that it was caused by a traumatic injury, the patient could drop out of the stroke quality measures and into the trauma registry.

Another factor that affects quality measures would be the severity of illness documentation, where inconsistencies could arise from physician documentation that is missing or sparse. Incomplete or limited details in physician documentation can result in a description of the problem that does not capture enough detail to code accurately. This type of problem could affect care coordination if the follow-up provider is unaware of the presenting issues or preclude necessary medical services ordered after the visit. It can also affect sampling for quality measures and the accuracy of mortality statistics.

Anatomy of the Coding Abstract

Every coding abstract has the same structure with vital patient information at the top, a summary of diagnosis codes, and a list of procedures by date at the bottom of the page. The entire coding abstract usually fits on a single printed page:

Patient Data
- Demographics (gender, age, race)
- Visit Dates
- Code Status
- Payor Type
- Discharge Disposition

Diagnosis Codes
- Admitting Diagnosis (A)
- Principal Diagnosis (P)
- All Other Secondary Diagnoses

Procedures By Date

The dates of the encounter (from admission to discharge), as well as other identifying patient information such as the discharge disposition are included at the top of the coding abstract. The suspected diagnosis from the initial medical assessment is called the "admitting diagnosis." The principal diagnosis code is what the physician documents as the over-arching problem that was treated during the encounter. It is the principal diagnosis code that usually pulls patients in and out of samples for quality measures. The other diagnosis codes are all the comorbidities, chronic conditions, and medical management codes that were also treated but were not the primary focus of the visit. These diagnosis codes also have indicators about whether the condition was Present On Admission (POA), as well as billing indicators based on the latest coding rules. Below the diagnosis codes are the procedure codes, including everything from bedside catheter insertions to major surgeries, along with the date of the procedure.

Another important detail to note is that inpatient codes come from an entirely different set of coding rules than outpatient codes. The codes are grouped by body systems (heart, brain, etc.), and providers try to be as specific as possible. Thankfully, every code with an accompanying translation of the abbreviations and a brief description of its meaning can typically be found with a quick web search, so unfamiliar codes do not often need expert consultation. However, an official review should be obtained for any discrepancies that affect sampling or abstraction.

The coding abstract is something to become comfortable reviewing because quality measures base population sampling on medical coding, and measure algorithms often contain reference tables with relevant diagnosis and procedure codes.

Ethics of Coding Reviews

There is a cautious ethical balance between holistic patient care and any review of the financial aspects of care found in coding and billing. Just as an abstractor should never abstract a chart inaccurately just to get a better score, a QI professional should not request coding changes to improve their metrics or to increase revenue.[1] Each facility will typically require some training about the ethical standards for this type of research, particularly about patient privacy and the ethics of reviewing financial reports on patient care, but it is worth repeating.

One respected authority in this area is the American Health Information Management Association (AHIMA), which publishes ethical standards for coding and documentation review. According to one of these ethical standards, the purpose of the review should always be to improve accuracy, not financial gain. Since quality measures affect reimbursement, the same ethical standards apply. AHIMA offers a variety of coursework on this topic, as well as others that may be of interest to a QI professional on their website.[2]

When in doubt, play it safe by adhering to the highest possible ethical standard and ask for feedback from the experts if there is any ethical question because violations of the professional ethical standards can have legal ramifications that could result in revocation of a license, financial penalties, or incarceration for fraud.[3]

Focus on Accuracy

So how does this review for accuracy in documentation affect QI? One important example is Mortality Review. When QI professionals start a diagnosis-specific Mortality Review, it keeps the focus on patient care and can reveal mismatches between reality and clinical documentation: If a patient dies from a bladder infection, the reviewer may wonder

1   The American Health Information Management Association (2016). Ethical Standards for Clinical Documentation improvement (CDI) Professionals. Retrieved Aug. 9, 2022, from https://bok.ahima.org/CDI_EthicalStandards.

2   The American Health Information Management Association (2022). Who We Are. Retrieved Aug. 9, 2022, from https://www.ahima.org/who-we-are/about-us/.

3   The Centers for Medicare and Medicaid Services (2022). Penalties. Retrieved Aug. 9, 2022, from https://www.cms.gov/regulations-and-guidance/administrative-simplification/enforcements/penalties/.

whether they had sepsis since most people survive bladder infections. If a patient dies from atrial fibrillation, the reviewer may question whether something else was going on since many patients live comfortably with medical treatment for atrial fibrillation.

Another occasion when coding may need to be reviewed is with the sampling of patient charts for abstraction. The rules for including and excluding patient charts for quality measure samples may change every six months, and there are often a few cases that need to have their coding reviewed due to conflicting information in the physician notes, or due to coding or specifications updates that do not yet flow effectively into the abstraction vendor tool. To continue with the brain injury example, abstractors for the stroke registry often need to clarify in the physician documentation whether a patient had a bleeding stroke, or whether the bleed was a complication from ischemic stroke treatment. These two different codes have vastly different results in care and reporting requirements. Another common example is when a patient has documentation of a prenatal complication from a clinic visit just prior to the hospital encounter and is then sent for an emergency cesarean section. On review of the chart at discharge, the admitting and operative notes may not mention the prenatal complications found prior to arrival due to the emergent nature of the visit, and the procedure could be coded as an elective surgery rather than an emergent intervention. These potential errors usually pop up when retrospective reviews are conducted, and the abstraction result is unexpected.

But how does a QI professional find these types of errors and anomalies, and what can be done about them? The first rule I learned is to never assume the worst, but to investigate thoroughly and gather any potential discrepancies for further review and discussion. The next section walks step-by-step through an example review. Although there is no pressure to follow them in order, the most common and easy-to-correct errors are listed first, and I found that it saved time to follow this process:

START WITH THE MANUALS

The specifications manuals are the primary tool for reviewing unexpected abstraction results or odd coding. The manuals are posted on their respective sites, so the CMS inpatient and outpatient manuals can be found on the CMS QualityNet website;[4] the Joint Commission manuals are also online;[5] and the AHA manuals are all available inside the AHA abstraction vendor tool online.[6] Some manuals are easier to use than others.

However, all the manuals use a coding algorithm to outline the standards of care and document the rationale for the measures. Following the logic-trail in the manuals is a lot like a flow chart. The coding algorithms include the rationale and guidelines, and they reveal why a patient should or should not be included in the population, or why the sampled chart passed/failed the measure. Every time I thought that I knew the specifications like the back of my hand, I would find some sentence or loophole that I had assumed meant one thing, only to discover it meant something else, and I would need to draw a new arrow in my mental flow chart. This initial review of the specifications manual is a great time to submit a clarification question to an expert, and each of the organizations that publish a manual have this option available online at their websites.

4   The Centers for Medicare and Medicaid Services (n.d.). QualityNet. Retrieved Sept. 10, 2022, from https://qualitynet.cms.gov/.

5   The Joint Commission (n.d.). Chart Abstracted Measure Specifications Manuals. Retrieved Oct. 27, 2022, from https://manual.jointcommission.org.

6   The American Heart Association (2015). Login. Retrieved Oct. 27, 2022, from https://heart.irp.iqvia.com.

VERIFY THE CODING ABSTRACT

The patient's coding abstract in the electronic medical record should be compared against the one in the vendor tool to see if there are any mismatches. This review is especially important after updates to the manual because there are times when the coding updates do not upload properly into the vendor tool. Other times, the coding is reviewed and updated after the vendor tool has uploaded an older version of the coding abstract, and an updated copy of needs to be submitted. These types of errors can be fixed fairly easily with an email or phone call to the vendor tool representative.

REVIEW THE DOCUMENTATION

Compare the patient's discharge summary and physician notes to the coding abstract to look for vague, sparse, or unclear documentation and/or missing documents. Sometimes there are notable differences in the record where the primary provider and the consulting provider have different conclusions, or there might be confusion about whether the patient had a chronic pre-existing condition or the sudden onset of a new condition. Other times, there is nothing worth mentioning because the documentation is clear.

If the specifications in the manuals are met, the coding abstracts agree, and the documentation is inclusive, the last option is to ask a colleague to take a second look. Otherwise, the unexpected result is likely correct, and an investigation of any missed opportunities can begin.

But if an error was found, several questions are bound to come up like: What happens next? Can anything be done to fix the error? What is the QI role when it comes to coding accuracy?

Clinical Documentation Integrity

Enter the Clinical Documentation Integrity (CDI) specialist. The CDI Department provides expert review for physicians, writes queries to the medical staff to clarify documentation, and reports to the Chief Financial Officer (CFO) at the facility. AHIMA states that CDI professionals ensure that events and services from the patient encounter are captured accurately in the medical record.[7] Again, the emphasis is on accuracy, not on revenue or metrics. And while AHIMA is geared to all health information management professionals, the Association of Clinical Documentation Integrity Specialists (ACDIS) provides certification standards and professional guidance specific to CDI specialists.[8]

To recap the process, coding is based on medical record documentation, and coding flows into quality reporting, reimbursement, and disease tracking. So the CDI specialist's scope of practice can influence coding accuracy, which affects QI projects.

The CDI specialist works under the CFO, and it is typical for the CFO to divide patients by insurance coverage. For example, the CDI professional could be asked to provide reports on the number of queries they send for Medicare beneficiaries with a specific diagnosis. Then they work with the physician to clarify documentation so that coding reflects the real patient picture and experience. One of the new topics gaining attention in the CDI world, as well as QI, is the importance of cooperation between these two departments: For the QI professional, the CDI specialist has a high level of knowledge about diagnosis codes and can help the QI professional avoid errors when requesting a coding review or documentation clarification.

Remember that there is a CMS rule that documentation cannot be

---

7   The American Health Information Management Association (n.d.). Who We Are. Retrieved Aug. 18, 2022 from https://www.ahima.org/who-we-are/about-us.

8   Association for Clinical Documentation Integrity Specialists (n.d.). Membership. Retrieved Aug. 18, 2022, from https://acdis.org/membership/mission.

altered in a medical record more than 30 days after the discharge date.[9] So working with the CDI specialist will not likely be about making corrections to charts before submission; rather, the focus should be on making corrections to the process that caused the error to occur in the first place. The CDI specialist can highlight areas of need by diagnosis, and the QI professional can work alongside medical staff to improve processes related to these areas of need, reducing the CDI workload of "problem cases" that require a query. For the CDI specialist, cooperation with QI can improve revenue recovery by lowering workloads, increasing documentation compliance, and most importantly, improving patient outcomes.

There are courses for CDI specialists to study quality measures and develop collaborative efforts, and the relationship between these fields continues to evolve. But keep in mind that not every facility has collaboration between the departments, and since QI reports to the clinical branch of administration and CDI reports to the financial branch, they probably do not have regular meetings or gather around the office water cooler to chat. However, getting to know your local CDI team and synergizing your departments will benefit both your quality scores and your hospital's bottom line. Bear in mind that your local CDI specialist has a heavy workload of detailed reviews, so it is critical to schedule a meeting time rather than drop by their workspace with random interruptions.

In my first facility, I collaborated with the facility CDI specialist, and we found our discussions so productive that we decided to meet regularly to discuss sepsis patients, obstetric procedure codes, and stroke diagnosis codes together. I also regularly discussed Mortality Review findings in these meetings to get a coding perspective on the severity of illness. During these discussions, we observed that we had patients in

---

9   The Code of Federal Regulations (2022). "Medicare Conditions of Participation: Medical Record Services." National Archives, 42 C.F.R. § 482.24 C(4)(viii). Retrieved March 18, 2022, from https://www.ecfr.gov/current/title-42/chapter-IV/subchapter-G/part-482.

Intensive Care who were intubated and receiving continuous vasopressor therapy, but the documented cause of death was something quite mild like bronchitis: There was clearly a mismatch between the severity of illness in reality, and the severity of illness in the documentation. As a QI professional, I found that appropriate care was given, but the documentation showed patients were dying from mild infections and it looked like poor-quality care. What was going wrong to have that kind of an outcome in mortality review?

I found that this problem actually originated with our new and improved rapid sepsis treatment protocol: Suddenly, patients looked better in a matter of hours compared to how they looked when they came in. With the new protocol, patients recovered while they were still in the Emergency Department, and the admitting physician was unaware of how sick they were on arrival. Ironically, our clinical improvements resulted in several problems. The flow of patient care looked something like this:

DAY I IN THE ED

- **PATIENT CONDITION:** Unresponsive, low blood pressure, tachycardia, kidneys shutting down, poor urine output, dry skin with a grayish-color, oxygenation decreasing slowly.

- **TREATMENT:** Fluid resuscitation, broad-spectrum IV antibiotics, mechanical ventilation with BiPAP, inserted Foley catheter, and frequent blood pressure monitoring.

- **ED DIAGNOSIS:** Weakness, tachycardia

In a few hours when the admitting physician visited, the situation had changed dramatically:

DAY I ON THE UNIT:

- **PATIENT CONDITION:** Alert and oriented, normal blood pressure, normal heart rate, good urine output, pink skin, nasal cannula, sitting up in bed eating lunch and asking if

---

they could go home.

- **TREATMENT:** Continue IV antibiotics, monitor blood pressure, discontinue Foley and prepare for discharge home in the morning.
- **DIAGNOSIS:** Bladder infection

The trouble with this situation is that the receiving care team had no idea that they needed to continue monitoring the patient's respiratory status, urine output, or kidney function, unless it was clearly documented and communicated to the receiving provider. In many cases, the patient's needs were obscured by vague or sparse documentation that described symptoms rather than a diagnosis. In addition, if the patient worsened, one of the negative habits that a physician could fall into is when the documentation for a previous note is carried over the next day without thorough review. Then, even if the patient's case became critical, the original diagnosis of "bladder infection" may be carried over rather than a diagnosis of severe sepsis with ongoing treatment. While this was a rare occurrence, we could tell that it frequently started in the ED handoff, and it could be continued through a process of poor documentation habits throughout the patient's stay.

After discovering these problems, our organization started a new program for CDI collaboration with QI to ensure that sepsis care was accurately reflected in the chart. We also worked with ED medical staff to document the severity of the patient's condition on arrival and clearly communicate with admitting physicians about the extent of sepsis treatments provided during the patient's ED encounter. We simplified sepsis templates for provider notes, and eventually, the admitting diagnoses of "weakness, tachycardia" occurred less often and were replaced by "r/o sepsis" and "severe sepsis without septic shock" after this collaboration.

These early interventions to improve documentation and communication with the team also resulted in nurses who could now see a more comprehensive report on the patient's problems. Now they could see where focused assessments of different body systems should occur to monitor progress with sepsis treatment. With the help of the ED

Medical Director, these efforts steered the ED physician role back to the diagnosis and treatment of patients rather than administrative tasks. Apparently, they had gotten pushback in the past about their problem statements from admitting physicians, but when we clarified the situation in medical staff committee presentations, the team was able to work together in a way that benefited patient care and reduced work for everyone. All of these benefits came from collaboration and a willingness to look deeper at a situation rooted in physician staff shortages and exhaustion to find a better solution for patients.

Informatics and Documentation Templates

Informatics professionals are key players in the healthcare team as every nursing assessment and physician template is reviewed, tested, and managed by them. For example, they were often able to figure out feasible documentation templates, order sets, and/or efficient workflows to pull patients by their diagnosis code. I am forever grateful for their patient willingness to help me solve project barriers. As I worked to become fluent with the review side of the medical record, I discussed the data that I needed to retrieve with the Informatics Department to see if I was using the most efficient method. Informaticists work with IT&S, but they are not in a traditional technical support role. Rather, they have a clinical role in IT&S, and they test any changes and updates to the electronic medical record to preview what it will be like for clinical staff to use it. When the changes are ready to go-live, they would send emails about how to use the updates. For someone who is unsure who to contact for their informatics questions, a good place to start is your email inbox: Just search for the last medical record update notification from your facility, and the author of that email usually knows who to contact for further information.

The informaticist could also tell me when an improvement request was not feasible because they are most familiar with the needs of a typical user. So, when I may have had personal preferences that others would not find helpful, the informatics professional could anticipate the user's needs and keep me on the right track. I met regularly with the informatics team and let them know what the end-goal was for each quality project, and I helped out with beta testing whenever they requested assistance. It is important to be patient when working on computerized documentation, though, because technical changes generally do not turn out well when rushed.

Although each step in the informatics world requires a lot of time and effort to set-up, it tends to reduce time and effort once it is launched. These projects require close, respectful collaboration with the informatics team. If I wanted to build a house, I would need a blueprint, collaboration with experts at each stage of construction, and even when the project is finished I would want to have it inspected for any hazards that may have been missed before I move in. Likewise, if I ask the informatics team to help me build a documentation template, I will spend time providing and reviewing drafts, collaborating with experts, and testing the template once it is built. It is well worth the effort, though, because it can increase efficiency and accuracy across multiple departments. Truthfully, a well-planned informatics project could increase efficiency for the entire hospital's workload by whole percentage points. Knowing that possibility exists, what exactly can a QI professional do to improve patient care through informatics?

Order Sets

Nobody likes order sets.

Physicians despise having an invisible "someone" that tells them what to do, nurses dislike the barrage of nursing orders in the sets because they are based on ideal situations, informaticists hate the level of detail requested by multiple sub-committees, and QI professionals despise reviewing them to ensure compliance with quality measures. They are nightmarishly tedious.

But order sets are wonderful for improving patient outcomes.

Order sets are pre-defined and based on evidence that actually works for patients, so it removes guesswork and reduces time spent looking up the best treatment for a *Clostridium difficile* infection, for instance. They help prevent errors of forgetfulness for the patient who arrives with a suspected heart attack, for example: Someone could have forgotten to order their heart medication until the discharge medication reconciliation, but with the admission order set, it was included automatically as an order prompt. Order sets can even provide a critical clue to diagnosis documentation—if the sepsis order set is used, then it follows that sepsis should likely be included in the problem list.

Early research findings show exciting results that the use of Computerized Physician Order Entry (CPOE) has the potential to reduce medical errors.[10] This is a big deal, because The Institute of Medicine set a national priority for reducing medical errors in their publication *To Err is Human*.[11] Further, in 2019 the CDC reported that unintentional injury was the third leading cause of death in the United States,[12] and a 2016 study in the British Medical Journal suggested that since there is no medical code for medical errors, that same "unintentional injury" measurement is perhaps the best capture of deaths caused by all medical errors.[13] To translate these findings: Medical errors are presumed to be the third leading cause of death in the U.S. So if the evidence supports the use of CPOE to reduce those medical errors, I will happily review order sets rather than deal with

---

10   Radley, D.C., et al (May 2013). Reduction in medication errors in hospitals due to adoption of computerized provider order entry systems. *J Am Med Inform Assoc* 20 (3): 470-6. Retrieved Aug. 7, 2022, from https://pubmed.nvbi.nlm.nih.gov/2345440/.

11   Kohn, L.T.; Corrigan, J.M.; Donaldson, M.S. (Eds.) (2000). *To Err is Human: Building a Safer Health System.* National Academies Press.

12   Heron, M. (2021). Deaths: Leading Causes for 2019. *National Vital Statistics Reports,* 70 (9): 18. Retrieved Oct. 27, 2022, from https://www.cdc.gov/nchs/data/nvsr/nvsr70/nvsr70-09-508..pdf.

13   Makary, M.S.; Daniel, M. (May 2016). Medical error – the third leading cause of death in the US. *BMJ,* 353: i2139. Retrieved Aug. 7, 2022, from https://www.bmj.com/content/353/bmj.i2139.

preventable patient harm afterwards.

In practice, I was responsible for reviewing each order on the new quality measure order sets. I needed to work with each department to review the orders for accuracy and feasibility. I met with the director of our laboratory to ensure a match with our lab practices, the CPOE pharmacist to verify the selected medications were available in the ordered form, and physician champions from the respective committees to make sure that everything met their unique clinical guidelines. Then I met with the informaticist to ensure that all of those details would be displayed clearly and correctly and that they resulted in the correct actions (like the labeling of lab specimens in response to a requisition order). I also followed patients around on the computer and spoke with the nurses and physicians to find errors in the digital workflow. Launching a new order set can take some time, but when our order set launched, it resulted in excellent provider-usage rates.

Once an order set is established, it should be reviewed at least annually to include updates from the specifications manuals or changes in the facility medication stock, for example. It is not a fun job, but I would caution that it is an important one that should not be neglected or signed off too quickly because timely maintenance is much easier than a total overhaul of a broken process.

Templates for Assessments

Documentation templates are another primary tool for reducing time spent on documentation. Rather than ask a provider to memorize the specifications manual, it is much more supportive to include the option of a template that matches the guidelines and prompts the provider to include the required material. For example, the facility might be able to create a heart failure discharge template with allowable contraindications to anticoagulant administration, rather than taking time from patient care to ask the physician if they did not order the anticoagulant because the patient was bleeding. Another good example would be the septic shock re-assessment, where each category is listed, and the lactate levels and vital signs are auto-populated.

These templates can be a wonderful tool for clinicians who do not want to be bothered about regulatory details or pressured to memorize a set of rules. However, any templates or printable materials should be reviewed at least annually to make corrections and updates, and physicians should be consulted before launching a physician template; as technology continues to evolve, consulting clinical users is still one of the best ways to keep the focus on feasible solutions for patients.

New Documentation Technology

HEALTH LEVEL SEVEN (HL7)

Did you know there is a federal policy on Health IT to develop national data exchange and interoperability? The dream is that a provider will be able to access previous patient encounters, even if the previous encounter occurred in a completely different medical record system. Hospital discharge paperwork could be immediately accessed by the primary care physician, and patients would not need to repeat their entire medical history with each new visit. And perhaps more important to QI professionals, this universal interoperability coupled with Artificial Intelligence technology could potentially result in automated data abstraction for even the most complex registries.

Now, I bet that got your attention!

In 2020, the National Coordinator for Health IT (ONC) announced the release of the **21st Century Cures Act: Interoperability, Information Blocking, and the ONC Health IT Certification Program Final Rule**, which set standards for safe and efficient access to the electronic health record.[14] These innovations are significantly led by an organization called **Health Level Seven International (HL7)**,[15] a non-profit accredited in standards development for clinical and administrative data. Their vision is for everyone in the world to have secure access to the right health data when they need it, and they provide standards to guide global health data exchange. One of the ways they are working to accomplish this goal is through the Fast Healthcare Interoperability Resources (FHIR) branch of the organization, which leads the charge on quick and efficient data exchange through application programming interface (API)-focused standards.[16] The major electronic medical record companies have voluntarily signed up to develop systems that can share data with each other while adhering to security and privacy standards based on the HL7 roadmap. So perhaps in the future, a pneumococcal given in Utah will be visible to the patient's provider in Vermont, even if the patient forgets when and where they got it.

But what about those Artificial Intelligence (AI) technologies I mentioned earlier? I would be remiss if I did not mention new technology that could affect the future of QI quite dramatically, and AI certainly has the potential to do so. Below are some examples that are currently in use:

- **SPEECH RECOGNITION DICTATION SOFTWARE**: A provider speaks into a microphone and the speech recognition software converts spoken words into written text in the chart.

---

14   Anthony, E. S. (March 9, 2020). The Cures Act Final Rule: Interoperability-Focused Policies that Empower Patients and Support Providers. *Health IT Buzz*. Retrieved Oct. 27, 2022, from https://www.healthit.gov/buzz-blog/21st-century-cures-act/the-cures-final-rule/.

15   Health Level Seven International (n.d.). Frequently Asked Questions. Retrieved Aug. 18, 2022 from http://www.hl7.org/about/faqs/.

16   The Office of the National Coordinator for Health Information Technology (n.d.). FHIR Fact Sheets. Retrieved Oct. 27, 2022, from https://www.heatlhit.gov/topic/standards-technology/standards/fhir-fact-sheets/.

- o Some providers are effectively dictating patient visits in real-time at their clinic, while AI scribes record and format the note for provider review.

- **DATA CRAWLERS**: The same technology used by search engines to suggests relevant websites based on keywords can also pull data from electronic patient charts.

  - o Electronic Medical Records are searchable, and search engine skills are transferable.

- **ARTIFICIAL INTELLIGENCE (AI) CLINICAL DECISION APPLICATIONS**: A computer program that gathers data and suggests possible diagnoses with roughly equivalent accuracy to a live provider.

  - o This technology is used by CDI specialists to improve query efficiency with specialized software.

  - o The first data abstraction companies are conducting AI-driven abstraction with human collaboration and IRR to verify accuracy. Over time, the computer "remembers" to avoid errors in future practice.

- **TELEHEALTH: TECHNOLOGIES**: These programs have innovated dramatically in the last few years due to the necessity of limited face-to-face interaction during the COVID-19 Pandemic for in-home visits and monitoring.

  - o Urgent care telehealth is now included with some insurance plans.

  - o Concierge medicine is gaining traction, where primary care services are provided based on a subscription model through primarily web-based service bundles rather than a fee-for-service on-site model.

  - o Emergency Rooms are hiring telehealth specialty services for rapid behavioral health evaluations to decrease excessive length of stay.

o   Neurologists can "visit" potential stroke patients and
    view their brain imaging from off-site to improve
    efficiency and accuracy with thrombolytic treatment
    decisions.

o   In-home counseling services have expanded the reach
    of addiction counseling and chronic symptom manage-
    ment.

o   In-home monitoring made hospital-at-home inpatient
    services possible during the COVID-19 Pandemic,
    because remote monitors could observe the patient and
    staff could easily upload vital signs.[17]

o   Some clinics use telehealth management for chronic
    conditions at-risk for readmission, reducing cost by
    providing in-home technician support for appoint-
    ments.[18]

o   Telesitters are utilized at some hospitals for monitoring
    patient rooms when the patient is at risk for falls. The
    sitter reports to on-site nursing staff if the patient is in a
    situation at-risk for injury.

17   Raths, D. (Sept. 14, 2022). Lessons Learned in ChristianaCare's Hospital at
Home Program. *Healthcare Innovation*. Retrieved Oct. 27, 2022, from https://
www.hcinnovationgroup.com/population-health-management/home-based-care/
article/21280709/lessons-learned-in-christianacares-hospital-at-home-program/.

18   Siwicki, B. (June 21, 2022). Telehealth with a technician in the home reduces
spend by 22% for Scottsdale Physician Group. *Healthcare IT News*. Retrieved Aug. 18,
2022, from https://www.healthcareitnews.com/news/telehealth-technician-home-re-
duces-spend-22-scottsdale-physician-group.

o   Facilities in Japan are using robots as nursing aids for basic duties, like lifting patients and helping them to use the toilet.[19]

I love efficiency, but I hate change. And I have noticed that as new technology emerges there seems to be a necessary balance between efficiency and information security: The most efficient methods are often the least secure, and the most secure methods are often the least efficient. Despite this concern, these technological advances could significantly affect the schedule and case load of healthcare professionals. Adaptations would need to be made in numerous aspects of healthcare, and each change would require measurement and evaluation at the local level, so these are topics that will certainly affect QI professionals.

Why are we even trying to integrate these new-fangled technologies into healthcare? Since many of these technologies could diminish staffing requirements, reduce wasted time, or open healthcare positions to global recruitment, we need to keep an eye on emerging technology and how it is implemented at pilot facilities. For instance, one hospital system recently implemented an AI-driven scheduling program to manage their staffing shortages.[20] Their precision staffing allowed managers to schedule the more than 10,000 nurses in their system up to 18 months in advance without over- or under-staffing. The program boasts improved predictability of facility needs because it is able to "see" six years of data and make predictions, rather than just looking at the previous year (which was quite unique after the COVID-19 Pandemic). They hope it will increase employee retention and patient satisfaction while allowing managers to provide more mentorship to inexperienced

19   Eggleston, K.; Suk Less, Y., et al (2021). Robots and Labor in the Service Sector: Evidence from Nursing Homes. *National Bureau of Economic Research*. Retrieved Nov. 1, 2022 from https://www.nber.org/papers/w28322.

20   Walker, C. (2022). Unique AI tool helps Sanford Health schedule nurses. *Sanford Health News*. Retrieved on March 18, 2022, from https://news.sanfordhealth.org/innovations/unique-ai-tool-helps-sanford-health-schedule-nurses/.

staff. Despite the AI system, individual managers retain the ability to make small changes to accommodate unique staffing needs. If this AI-driven staffing program is effective, it could cut a veritable mountain of hours from the management team's scheduling workload.

These types of "disruptive" technologies could affect the national labor shortage. Since workforce shortages are reaching critical levels according to the American Hospital Association (AHA), I believe this need might be the final push for significant digital integration in health-care.[21] Telehealth and AI have the ability to improve access to quality care for our most vulnerable patients; but telehealth and AI also have the potential to completely obscure the needs of our most vulnerable patients. As QI professionals, we need to actively discuss and investigate new technology and examples of digital transformation.

During any discussion of change, it is important to share both the difficulties and potential improvements to the electronic record with the whole healthcare team—no one should be left in the dark amidst such dramatic changes. That means discussions about "how we always used to do things" must happen without condescension, and openness to change will come hand-in-hand with an openness to listen to the needs of patients and professionals. The Quality Department will surely be involved in such changes to ensure that quality is maintained in patient care as the facility navigates such changes. There is a difference between intelligence and wisdom, and the future of our field will need to combine Artificial Intelligence with real-life wisdom and compassion.

---

21   American Hospital Association (Nov. 1, 2021). Fact Sheet: Strengthening the Health Care Workforce. Retrieved on March 18, 2022, from https://www.aha.org/fact-sheets/2021-05-26-fact-sheet-strenghtening-health-care-workforce.

Chapter 7
Conclusions

The Quality Improvement Role

One of the things that I was afraid to lose when I moved from bedside nursing to the administrative wing was the team atmosphere and consistent support from peers. I love how nurses help each other with unstable patients, settling new admissions, picking up each other's lunches, and offering support during emotionally draining times. I grieved inwardly when I left my team in the ICU because I believed that I would be much more alone in my new desk job. Despite those fears, I still felt like it was a good fit for my skill set, and I committed to make the best of it.

However, when I moved into an analyst job, I discovered a diverse team of professionals would be working with me. I found people that were willing to hear my ideas and offer feedback, help me find resources, and who were eager to share their own ideas and innovations with me. We solved problems together and helped each other with a variety of diverse tasks, covered each other's vacations by cross-training, and brainstormed together on our toughest problems. Another surprise was that I was able to stay connected to colleagues within my region who were sorting through the same problems that I was facing. Finally, by participating in conferences and online forums, I made connections with QI professionals across the country who were eager to discuss innovative approaches to the same problems that I was facing.

If you feel alone or lost in the QI world, please know that there are others willing to support and mentor you, as well as hear your innovative ideas and fresh perspective. Each of the organizations discussed in this book have opportunities to connect in some way, whether through professional conferences, webinars, or online forums. Also, do not be shy about cold-calling other professionals or vendor representatives who seem knowledgeable.

Because we believe so strongly in helping each other improve patient care, PorterQI© offers a podcast titled *Quality for the Rest of Us*, to share stories from professionals like you and reveal clever solutions to the healthcare mysteries we all face. PorterQI.com also offers an online community with fresh resources and a social site for professionals to connect and improve in a supportive environment.

Wherever you find your supportive team, remember to pass on the knowledge and skills you acquire to the people who are new to the field so that we can build on the legacy given to us and improve the lives of our patients.

In the words of Helen Keller, "**Together we can do so much.**"[1]

---

1   Adams, K. (June 26, 2018). "Helen Keller: 'Alone We Can Do So Little, Together We Can Do So Much.'" American Foundation for the Blind Blog. Retrieved March 18, 2022, from https://www.afb.org/blog/entry/happy-birthda-helen.